# A HARD LESSON WASTED

## The Bahamas Cholera Epidemic

Harold A. Munnings

eBook ISBN 978-976-8205-67-4

Paperback ISBN 978-976-8205-64-3

# Contents

# Acknowledgements

The Bahamas Department of Archives takes its responsibility for the care of our valuable national archives seriously. I thank its staff for their professional assistance with accessing the records so essential to my research.

Many of our valuable primary sources are held overseas, in the British National Archives. I am grateful to the archivists there for fulfilling my requests for information and to the librarians of the Latin American & Caribbean Collection Digital Newspaper Library of the University of Florida George Smathers Library. I thank Katie Birkwood, the Rare Books and Special Collections librarian at the Royal College of Physicians of London, for her help with information on the Farre family of physicians, and Mr Peter Henderson, the archivist at the King's School in Canterbury, and Danielle Spittle and Stephen Willis from the University of Edinburgh Centre for Research Collections for information on Governor Gregory's early education. I thank the Library of the College of Charleston Special Collections, the South Carolina

Historical Society Archives and the Librarians of the South Carolina Room of Charleston County Public Library for the material on the *Ovando* emigrants after they left the Bahamas. I thank Amy Ackerman at the Main Library of St Augustine, Florida and Charles Tingley of the St Augustine Historical Society for their help during my visit, as I pursued Talbot Bethell's report that cholera was brought to the colony from that ancient city in Florida. I thank Jim Lawlor for his encouragement, his perspectives on Governor Gregory and for his permission to quote from *Harbour Island Story*. I thank the Anglican Diocese of The Bahamas and the Turks and Caicos Islands and The Bahamas Conference of the Methodist Church for permission to access their church archives, and I thank Ms Sonja Balfour and Pastor Bill Higgs and Ms Meggan Lightbourne for facilitating my request.

If there is an aspect of Bahamian history on which Captain Paul Aranha does not have some picture or lead, I have yet to encounter it. I thank my friend for the images he shared of the New Providence neighbourhood where cholera first broke out, and of the St Matthew's Burial Ground, retrieved from his immense personal collection. I thank Ann Morley-Carmel, expert Bahamian genealogist, for the information that she provided on multiple personalities who were a part of my story of this epidemic. I thank Eric Wiberg, The Bahamas' premier nautical historian, for information about the vessels in the story and for helping me to understand the Victorian-era transatlantic and regional colonial transportation system. I thank Dwayne Archer of the Department of Statistics, and Dr Blair Woodside of the Department of Epidemiology, for their assistance with the nation's statistics that helped provide a perspective of the impact of cholera. I thank Robert Deal, general manager of the Water and Sewerage Corporation, for his permission to access the Corporation's historical records, and Dr Richard Cant, veteran hydrologist and cataloguer of the Corporation's records, and Michael Swann, the Corporation's historian, for the documents that detailed the slow march to the introduction of the capital's waterworks.

I am fortunate to enjoy the friendship of Virginia Ballance, University of The Bahamas Health Sciences librarian and an expert in digital scholarship. Her Internet search skills have been in constant service of this project. Its quality was also significantly elevated by the critique gratefully received from Dr Rita Pemberton, retired head of the Department of History at UWI St Augustine and from Dr Grace Turner, archeologist and expert on Bahamian burial grounds, who also kindly shared Henry Stevenson's unique first-hand account of the epidemic.

Portions of this cholera story have been shared with The Bahamas Historical Society and on the radio as my research progressed. I am grateful to the organisers for the public platforms they provided, which revealed the interest in the story that exists in the community. I thank my son, Harry, for graphing the Board of Health's epidemic statistics; my brilliant niece, Gabrielle Gweneth Misiewicz, for paring and ordering the story; my draft readers Anthony Munnings and Patricia Collins, who identified areas that needed clarification and correction; Victoria Sarne, draft editor and copyeditor, Dan Shutt. Finally, I thank Jennifer, my daughter, herself a social scientist, for cheering me on, and Moneira, my wife, who understood, better than did I, how much this would take.

# List of Illustrations and Images

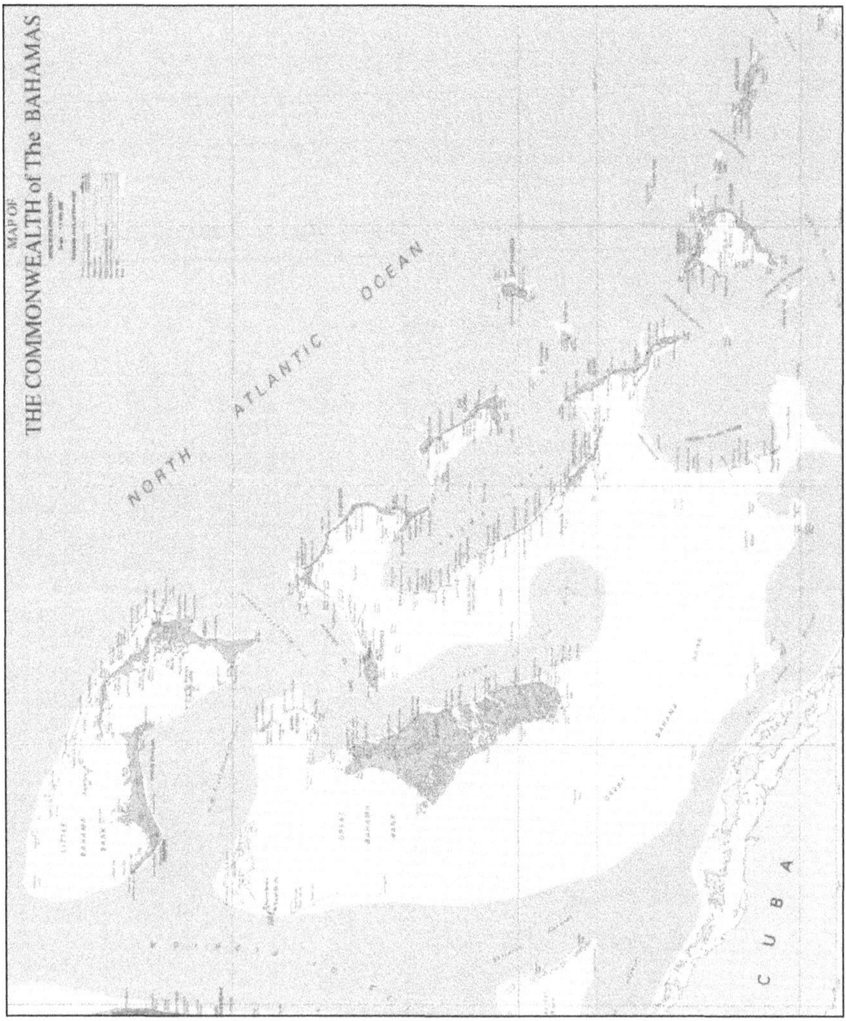


*1. Map of The Bahamas. Courtesy of the Department of Lands and Surveys, The Bahamas*

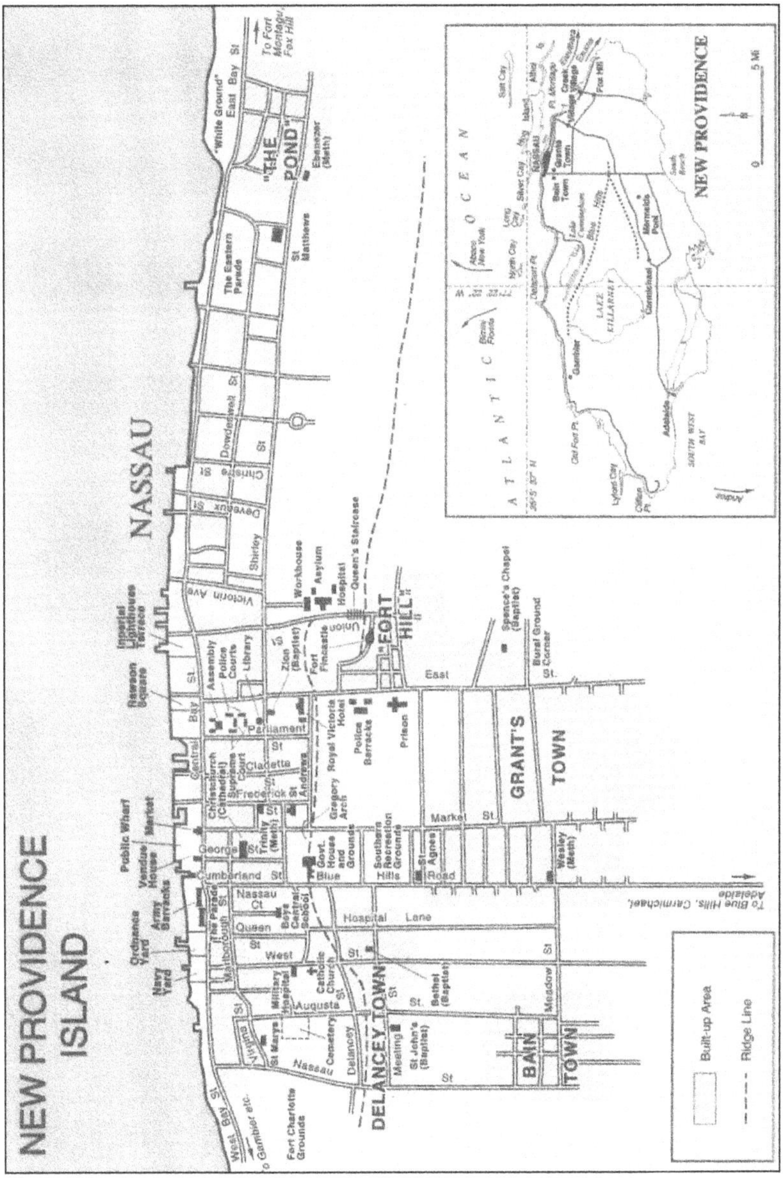


*2. Map of Nassau/New Providence, 1891*

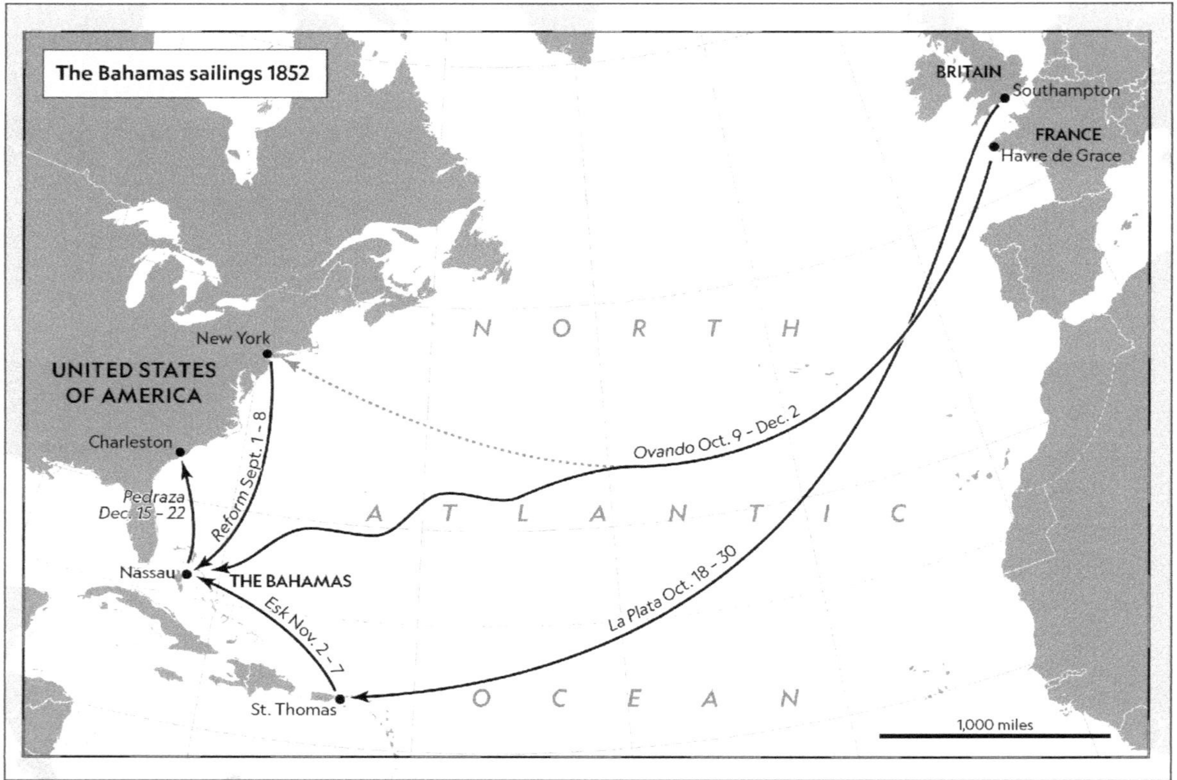


*3. Key sailings to and from The Bahamas, 1852*

# Introduction

In a contest of the most lethal events in the history of the people of The Bahamas, the cholera epidemic of 1852 holds the chilling second-place trophy. After the decimation of the Lucayans by the colonisers who followed Columbus, nothing has killed as many people in as short a period of time as the cholera epidemic. This is the story of that disaster.

Considering how well the epidemic was documented as it unfolded, it is a wonder that this work is the first to explore it in any detail. Craton's *History of The Bahamas* (1968), where I first heard of the epidemic, dispensed with it in just two sentences. *Islanders in the Stream* (1998), a large two-volume history of The Bahamas, covered it on a single page. My deep dive began when the lockdowns that attended the onset of the Covid-19 epidemic forced me to stay at home. I mined *The Nassau Guardian* and the *Bahama Herald* for reportage. Craton was not exaggerating when he wrote that a complete history of The Bahamas since 1844 could be written just from the files of *The Nassau Guardian*. It carried the votes of the Assembly, the laws, government accounts and statistical and other official reports. Available on microfilm since the 1970s, in 2020 access and readability improved dramatically when the University of Florida digitised the collection and made it available online.

When The Bahamas Department of Archives reopened to the public, I unearthed more of the cholera story from its records. Minutes of the Executive Council (see Appendix 6) documented the colony's response from within the administration. The decades-old microfilms were practically unreadable and I was most grateful that the chief archivist granted me access to the original books. I twitched in my chair as the giant volumes were placed on the reading room table and I was handed a pair of gloves. On my first day in possession of those fragile records, written when my great-grandfather Henry Alexander Munnings was two years old, I spent too many minutes gazing at the flawless and artful penmanship. My allotted time was almost up before I snapped out of the spell and began to take notes. My research was completed just in time as, owing to the brittle condition of some pages, the archivist closed the books for good.

Additional information was located in the British National Archives and in various libraries. In professional journals, I found letters written by doctors on the scene, who described their work and gave their opinions. Valuable information was found in church and military reports, in the pages of out-of-print books and pamphlets and even in New Providence graveyards. At the library of the St Augustine Historical Society in Florida, I followed up on what turned out to be a false lead on the origin of the epidemic. In the special collections of the South Carolina Historical Society, I found evidence of the fate of emigrants from Europe who passed through the colony at the height of the epidemic. The various sources painted a picture of the political, medical and social aspects of the disaster. I gained a glimpse of how the colony was run and exposed shortcomings, some of which shackled the colony's development for the next century.

Governor John Gregory sits at the centre of that core of remarkable personalities who headed the epidemic response. His name lives on in The Bahamas through Gregory's Arch, the gateway to Grants Town adjacent to Government House, and in Gregory Town, Eleuthera. However, a defining period of his administration was the cholera epidemic. Charles Nesbitt, the colonial secretary, was Gregory's key man before, during and after the event. The skills that made him so valuable to the string of governors he served were on full display during the epidemic. Chief among the health professionals practising at the time were Horatio Nelson Chipman, Frederick Duncome and William Kirkwood. The epidemic story revealed individual strengths that they employed in the service of the community, as well as weaknesses that, by the standards of today, seem trifling.

The natural consequence of consulting the written record is that the narrative is drawn primarily from the leadership. The voice of the working Bahamian is harder to perceive, but I have tried to share something of their experience. The event hit them the hardest as it went on to set records for mortality. They are visible in the population statistics and in the utilisation of the healthcare resources provided by the government. Special attention was paid to the workings of the Board of Health and its public pronouncements on cholera, which were aimed at the working man. Formed only two years before the epidemic, this body led the fight, with the aid of the local medical men, with whom it had turbulent relations. The doctors named and discussed the first victim; the modern code of protecting an individual's identity was not followed with any rigor in the 1850s. This enabled me to trace her activity and whereabouts when she fell ill. The spread of the epidemic through New Providence and to the Out Islands was tracked, helped by the weekly statistics released by the Board of Health.

Cholera had struck Jamaica before it reached The Bahamas. The epidemic there caused the Colonial Office in London to appoint the British Empire's first West Indies medical inspectors. Hector Gavin, the restless and undiplomatic appointee who came to New Providence, was perhaps the most entertaining of the personalities in The Bahamas cholera saga. He arrived with solid credentials and with the goodwill of the governor. As a consequence, he enjoyed free rein early on, but his hyperactivity proved impossible to reel in when he went beyond his brief. Had his terms of service been more strictly defined, he might have avoided the ugly clash at the end. Had he been more diplomatic and politically savvy, he might have made a lasting positive impact on the health of the colony. As it happened, the indifferent and tight-fisted government tossed the health initiatives that he had promoted, leaving the poor no better off after the epidemic than they had been before. And the epidemic gave them a taste of how vulnerable their civil rights, such as the right to privacy, were to attack. The Board of Health's house-to-house visitors' programme cancelled their right to privacy in their homes, and they relinquished control of their bodies if they were admitted to the cholera hospital. How the disease was managed there is described, as is the struggle with burials, the role of race and the Church, and a Baptist Minister's run-in with the government that blew up into an embarrassing debacle.

*A Hard Lesson Wasted* draws to a close with a description of the aftermath, when the colony counted the cost of the disaster in lives lost and in pounds, shillings and pence. The administration was soon distracted as one emergency after another the hit the colony in quick succession, including the wreck of the *William and Mary* and the death of the governor himself. It never got around to conducting an assessment of the disaster. The lessons that would have been contained in a report on the event might have served as a valuable guide for the management of future epidemics. How and why it was so soon forgotten is explored, and I show how forgetting caused the colony to fall behind its regional fellows.

Through all the remarkable discoveries made during my cholera investigations, most striking were the similarities between it and the recent Covid-19 pandemic. For instance, in both, The Bahamas was caught in a pandemic that swept in from Asia. In both, treatments initially hyped as life-saving were found to be ineffective and sometimes harmful. In both, governments issued chafing decrees that proved impossible for everyone to follow. In both, the authorities adopted emergency powers and discovered that loopholes in the emergency orders were exploited for gain.

Communities suffer secondary harm after a disaster, when resources allocated for relief and recovery are siphoned off, diverted or hoarded. Governments have to balance the need for a rapid response with the risk of losing control of money and supplies. Disaster planning has to include a robust system of checks and oversight to mitigate this problem. The conversations that led to the beginnings of such a system in The Bahamas could have started as early as 1853, but the government never took in the lessons of the cholera epidemic. The experience of terror, conflict and desperation it caused presents a cautionary tale for those who administer national resources in a time of disaster. In the pages that follow, I describe the hard lesson that the epidemic served the colony 170 years ago, and how it went to waste.

# 1

## Victorian New Providence

In the sweltering heat of July 1852, swarms of ants appeared from nowhere in Bain and Grants Town. In places, masses of them covered the road, making it impossible to walk without crunching hundreds underfoot with every step. Armies of ants invaded yards, attacking lizards, blinding hogs and biting people.

To many old-timers, the swarms were an ominous sign that disease could be near. Henry Farre, a visiting Englishman, saw the swarms for himself. He waved off the fears of the elders as the imaginings of an ignorant and superstitious people.[1] Farre was a man of science and scientists watched the weather. Changes in rainfall, temperature and humidity were believed to be indicators of the risk of fevers and disease. Laymen were more attuned to changes in animal behaviour and in the Victorian era swarms of pests had been linked to an approaching cholera epidemic.[2] The possible association between pests and disease was nothing new – plagues of frogs and insects had been known to precede epidemics since biblical times.[3]

On September 16, 1852, two months after the swarms of ants were sighted, cholera appeared in New Providence. It struck on the other side of town, in a picturesque suburb opposite the Eastern Parade. Its first victim was an affluent White woman and her death shocked the community. Immediately there were questions: How did she get it? Where had she been? Who was the man that she had visited in the days before she had fallen ill?

❦ ❦ ❦

On the evening of April 1, 1824, Kate lay on her back with a midwife standing at her side. Attendants fetched water and mopped beads of sweat from Kate's brow. Every few minutes, her teeth clenched, her head tossed and her face contorted with yet another futile contraction. She was weak after hours in labour. The Black granny had done her best but Kate's birth canal was just not big enough for the baby. By 8 p.m., the infant was dead and Kate herself was approaching a dangerous state. Word reached the Honourable Patrick Brown that Kate, his house slave, would probably not survive the night. He sent for Dr Tynes, who, recognising a complex problem that might be beyond his ability, sent for Dr Townsend to assist. Townsend slipped away from a dinner party at the home of the chief justice to meet his colleague at Mr Brown's estate.

In the nineteenth century, anyone could set up shop and practise medicine in The Bahamas. With no fixed educational or licensing requirements, from a legal standpoint, the university-trained physician, the bush doctor and the granny were on an equal footing. Not until the passage of the Bahamas Medical Act of 1906 was there even a formal register of practitioners.[4] The dearth of doctors and the valuable service that informally trained healers provided had forced the government to acknowledge this practical reality in the Act. It allowed for the licensure of individuals who had not obtained a medical diploma but who were 'possessed of skill in medicine or surgery'.[5] Clergy and Out Island commissioners were the main licensees under this Act, but there were others, including Evans Cottman, the former school biology teacher who wrote the classic memoir *Out Island Doctor*. However, diploma-toting medical professionals were the only healers that the government would employ, and they were the only ones trusted by colonialists. They were all White men, naturally, and steeped in the European school of thought. This meant that their remedies were, in the main, unpleasant. They blistered the skin, on the principle that this drew poisonous agents to the surface, and they bled patients to rid the body of imagined poisons. They induced diarrhoea and vomiting to rebalance a body's disturbed chemistry and they prescribed toxins like mercury and the narcotic opium for almost everything, including to treat cholera.[6]

The capabilities of doctors formally trained in Europe and America varied greatly, as did those of native healers and grannies. White citizens generally believed that Black 'bush' doctors were ignorant, but they were mistaken. Among native healthcare workers throughout the Caribbean could be found expert African-born healers. Some of the Igbo, who were taken from south-eastern Nigeria, and the Yoruba, from present-day Togo and Benin, had undergone apprenticeships lasting years. The plants they encountered as slaves were new to them, but they had plant literacy. Guided by characteristics such as smell, colour, leaf arrangement and habitat, skilled healers could identify similarities and point to those plants of potential medicinal value. This led to the development of a new and effective local pharmacopeia that was passed down by oral tradition.[7]

The prejudice of the White citizenry denied them the benefits of medicines available to Black people. However, notwithstanding their toxic and sometimes comical medical interventions, a White doctor with surgical skills, like those Townsend possessed, could make a world of difference. Peter Solomon Townsend had himself been unwell when he came to New Providence in December 1823. Having escaped the cold of New York for his own health's sake, he recovered after a period of rest, with visits to the beach and a diet of local fruit. It was not a total holiday; he had travelled with his instruments and had recently started a local practice when Tynes called for his help. On examining Kate, he confirmed the midwife's assessment that her baby was dead. Her only hope of surviving was for a swift delivery. Townsend perforated the infant's skull and removed its brain, making it possible for the stillborn to be delivered.

One may have hoped that this was the end of Kate's ordeal, but it was not. Her weakened uterus failed to expel the placenta – a problem that complicates some deliveries, especially after prolonged labour. Townsend removed it manually, and Kate endured this without the benefit of anaesthesia, asepsis or antibiotics, as is routine today. He then dashed to the home of Mr Wildgoose on Bay Street, who was in pain from an inability to pass urine. Townsend found that he was suffering from a urethral stricture and catheterised him, providing instant relief.

Before returning to New York near the end of the year, Townsend would operate on another slave girl for pterygium (a fleshy overgrowth of the membrane on the surface of the eye) and perform complex oral surgery on a seven-year-old child. He encountered a quack or two during his stay, but the astonishing instances of care that he and doctors like him rendered bolstered the stature of trained health professionals in the community.

We will never know whether he managed to save Kate's life. There was nothing more of her in his diary, which found its way to The Bahamas Historical Society more than a century later.[8] It is likely that she died of infection, but she may have survived. Townsend gave her a chance.

❦ ❦ ❦

For a long time after Townsend's departure, the colony lacked a skilled resident surgeon. From time to time, the absence would be sorely felt, as it was in New Providence one Sunday in December 1849. A nine-year-old girl was at home in the Eastern District playing with a tobacco pipe when she accidentally inhaled the stem. It lodged in her trachea, blocking her windpipe. The child struggled to breathe as three doctors tried in vain to remove the obstruction. None of them was able to perform a lifesaving tracheotomy and, after twelve hours of agony, the child died.[9]

A few months later, on Wednesday, March 26, 1850, a long dry spell in New Providence was broken by the onset of pouring rain. The downpours continued for four days and then, on the morning of March 29, the skies became foreboding, with thick black clouds covering the sky. The barometer fell and, around noon, torrential rain began to fall. Somewhere over that uninhabited swath of the island in the south-west known as the Pine Barrens, a twister formed. The spiral built into a full-blown tornado as it descended to threaten the rock, pine and palm trees that inhabited the Barrens, which even seventy years later was still referred to as a 'commercially valueless' wasteland.[10]

Grants Town is a low-lying community on flat ground that spreads southward on the other side of the long limestone ridge that separates it from the town of Nassau. It began as a squatter's community of free Blacks and, in 1825, Governor Lewis Grant had the surveyor-general formally lay out the settlement. Lots were sold to those workers who serviced the town of Nassau.[11] After Emancipation, it grew rapidly with an influx of formerly enslaved persons who were now market vendors and maids, stevedores and labourers.[12] Among its residents were capable blacksmiths, masons and carpenters, and some owned petty shops that sold homegrown fruit and vegetables. In the 1840s, Bain Town sprang up at the district's western border. By 1850, Grants Town had its own market and together both communities came to be called Over-the-Hill.[13]

On that morning of March 29, the tornado that had formed over the Barrens missed the wasteland and touched down in Bain Town. From there it began a north-eastward trek, tearing up everything in a strip thirty yards wide that stretched through Grants Town and continued all the way to East Bay Street.[14] It flattened walls, shredded houses and uprooted the strongest trees. St Agnes Church was damaged and the massive wall and northern gate of the New Providence Asylum was toppled.[15] The cyclone seemed to have strengthened as it approached the waterfront and on Bay Street it demolished George Millar's stone building and blacksmith forge.[16]

The mayhem of howling wind, the gunshot-like sound of beams cracking and the ballistic hazard of flying missiles was all over in a matter of minutes. In its wake came the sound of groans and cries from amid the rubble. The island's doctors dashed to the scene and among the first to arrive was Dr Chipman.

Horatio Nelson Chipman was born in 1804 in the waterfront township of Cornwallis, Nova Scotia. Named after Britain's greatest admiral, he was a teenager when his family moved to The Bahamas. Charles, his father, sent him to the University of Edinburgh. Medical diploma in hand, the young doctor returned to Nassau to practise. A former Member of Parliament who would soon be nominated to the Legislative Council, Chipman was now the most senior of the tiny local medical fraternity. He co-owned an important private pharmacy, the Apothecaries Hall, which was attached to his clinic on Frederick Street. The year before the tornado, he had decided to slow down a little and had given up his public duty as superintendent of the New Providence Asylum. In its place, he became the medical attendant to the African Hospital.[17]

Chipman rescued little Miss Mary Bassett from the wreckage of a home. Seven persons had been crushed to death or mortally wounded by flying debris, including George Hield, the sexton of St Agnes; Lewis Wood and his three children; and Samuel Dean. Dozens crawled out from under wreckage, including twenty people who were badly injured. Reverend Woodcock, curate of St

Agnes, opened his schoolhouse to be used as a field hospital. There, Dr Clutsam used his coat to make a sling for a woman with a broken arm, while others were tended by Dr Black, Dr Duncome and a Dr Taylor.[18]

In the afternoon, Governor Gregory, Archdeacon Trew and other bigwigs visited the scene and were moved by the sight. The injured slept at the schoolhouse and the following morning Chipman had them moved to the African Hospital, minus Rosette Fernander, who had died that evening of her injuries.[19]

A commission was quickly formed to estimate the property losses and to identify any persons with urgent needs. Grants Town was clearly the hardest hit, the scene of all of the fatalities and with fifty-eight residents suddenly homeless. The commission counted 105 buildings destroyed and tabulated the damage at £4,480. 'Only' thirty-one of the homes lost were in the Eastern District, the remainder being in Bain, Grants and Delancey Towns. In a rare departure from the norm of ignoring Black people unless they had been convicted of some offence, the commission had the names of all of those who had lost their homes published in the press.[20]

Material relief efforts began, as in every disaster, with the actions of neighbours and friends. Mr Weech opened a Tornado Relief Fund at his store and was appointed the custodian for donations of cash as well as clothing, bedding and furniture. Special collections were taken at church and Clutsam gave a public lecture at which a donation was collected for the Fund. His topic, 'The Advantages of Education', must have been a soothing balm for this intended audience. Black residents were mostly illiterate, and not entirely by choice. The House of Assembly created its own disaster fund and voted for a £700 contribution, amounting to approximately 15 per cent of the calculated damage and representing less than the salary of the chief justice. The Imperial Government pledged a matching grant.

The governor appointed a separate commission to allocate and distribute the mean aid. Its members were familiar figures in the circle of the colony's decision-makers: Felix MacCarthy, John Ferguson Cooke and Thomas Mathews, all White members of the Executive Council. William Henry Doyle, a White Bahamian barrister, and John Saffery George, a merchant, were also appointed. It lacked a single representative from Bain or Grants Town.[21]

In the same edition of the *Guardian* that announced the committee, a letter appeared that pointed out that not only poor Black citizens had suffered. The chief justice had reportedly lost valuable furniture and the Honourable Hugh Kerr had lost 'several of his houses'. Benjamin Bethel and William H. Fulford claimed to have suffered £800 in damage between them. The missive may well have been a well-intended effort to balance the record, but its timing suggests that someone was preparing the way for affluent friends, who may have had an eye on the relief money.

Overall, the community's response to this disaster is instructive. As always, private citizens rushed in to help in advance of the government. The snap creation of a first-aid centre showed quick thinking, with the medical community having upheld the high tenets of the profession's ancient oath. The colony's leadership began with genuine concern for the poor, but its allocation of relief was mean and its committees were devoid of any representation from Grants Town. There is a real possibility that some of the aid earmarked for those most in need was diluted or in part diverted.

The tornado disaster sent a clear message that the government was unprepared for a mass-casualty event. It ought to have provoked a discussion about how best to prepare for another disaster, such as a hurricane or an epidemic, but no such conversation took place. The tornado lesson went totally to waste.

❦ ❦ ❦

On the evening of January 9, 1851, the sound of a child in agony pierced the quiet of a night in Grants Town.

In the wake of Emancipation, Grants Town had rapidly expanded into a close-knit community. Many houses shared a common yard, as they do to this day. Everyone in the vicinity could tell that the howling was coming from the home of Mr Weech. His daughter, who had been fine at supper and had gone to bed without a fuss, was sobbing. She had abruptly awoken, clutching her abdomen and groaning. Her distress seemed to be worsening by the minute.

In the 1850s, a range of diseases sickened children in the colony that today are prevented by vaccines, proper sanitation and a healthy diet. The Board of Health published the sorry list for all to see; of the 252 deaths that occurred in the first half of 1852, fifty were killed by 'fever' (20 per cent) and twenty-five by tuberculosis (10 per cent).[22] Five children were lost to 'teething', a now-obsolete term for a condition that presented with fever and fits, and which was probably meningitis.[23] In the same period, eighteen children died from dysentery and two from whooping cough.[24] However, the greatest number of deaths by far, 112 (44 per cent), fell under a category labelled 'other'.[25] Today, this category accounts for 39 per cent of all deaths, but in only 1 per cent is the cause unknown.[26] I strongly believe that many of the ill-defined deaths in 1852 were the direct or indirect result of pellagra.

In the nineteenth century, pellagra was the most prevalent vitamin deficiency disease in the Americas. It was so common in the south-eastern United States that in 1914 the Spartanburg Pellagra Hospital opened in South Carolina to treat this one disease. In The Bahamas, it put more people in hospital than did alcoholism and caused more hospital deaths than tuberculosis.[27] Pellagra is caused by a lack of the B-vitamin niacin (vitamin B3) and presents with diarrhoea, a scaly rash and mental disturbances that can range from forgetfulness and depression to full-blown psychosis.[28] Even when the distinctive symptoms of pellagra are absent, a deficiency of niacin makes the body vulnerable to other diseases. The poor man's diet of grits, roots and pigeon peas was deficient in this vitamin. Many of Mr Weech's neighbours in Grants Town would not have been able to afford the niacin-rich chickens or eggs they produced for sale in the market.

Children had to survive vitamin deficiencies and infectious diseases to live to adulthood. For a family at the base of the colony's social pyramid, this was a major challenge. In 1852, the *Bahama Herald* described 'the so-called houses' in Grants Town as 'Unfit for dog kennels'.[29] Families slept crowded together in ramshackle and suffocating one-room dwellings. Cooking and defecation took place in the yard. The outside toilet, or privy, was a dilapidated wooden shack, thrown together with gaps in the planks that allowed snakes into the warm enclosure. Just enough light streamed in to allow for a glimpse of the critters that infested the walls of the hole. The scent that emanated from the shacks and from nearby piles of uncollected garbage attracted hordes of flies. Curious tourists explored the area from time to time, and later they came with photographers in tow. They disregarded the privation and composed quaint scenes of seemingly cheerful poverty.[30] Reverend Woodcock, the Anglican schoolmaster and the English minister of the town Methodist chapel would have been among the few White people who were regulars of Grants Town. Others generally avoided the Over-the-Hill area, and, naturally, no trained doctors lived or practised there. Its residents would have welcomed the attention of the same men who cared for the elite. But White doctors' fees were high and, after Emancipation, a personal expense. Only a major crisis could make a Black man contemplate spending that kind of money.

On that fateful January night in Grants Town, a bush doctor was at hand. A medicinal tea was prepared, but the little girl could not stomach any drink. Her groaning turned to wailing, and when she began to retch and vomit, Mr Weech realised that he could lose her. The question of money fell away and the only problem became who to call. Which physician would leave his home at this hour to rush to the home of a Black labourer in Grants Town? In a demonstration of astonishing insight, Weech knew exactly where to turn.

A messenger was dispatched. He took off straight up Market Street, the most direct route to Nassau. Chipman was nearest. He lived on the corner of Princes and Market Street, literally at the doorstep of Grants Town. His practice and public duties were well known. Word may have leaked that he was not happy that former governor Mathew had cut his stipend for working at the African Hospital. His request for it to be restored would shortly be excoriated by the editor of the *Bahama Herald*, who would call for the doctor (and any other civil servant who was not happy with their pay) to simply resign.[31] There was also talk that Chipman had a secret arrangement with another doctor that kept him covered in case the government decided to close the African Hospital. The record certainly supported the sip-sip that he kept an eye on the dollar.[32]

The messenger bypassed Chipman. Some may have guessed that he was headed to Cascadilla, the two-story mansion on East Street that was the home of William Kirkwood. As far as physicians went, he was the colony's top dog. Kirkwood was born in Belfast, but he grew up in New York.[33] He gained his medical diploma from the University of Pennsylvania, then America's oldest and most highly regarded medical school.[34] Its entire curriculum was a course of nineteen weeks of lectures, with no practical or bedside teaching. Graduates generally sought a hospital position or joined up with an established physician before venturing out on their own.[35] The most diligent furthered their education in Europe. Kirkwood went to Paris and then returned to New York to practise, where he fell ill with what appears to have been tuberculosis. In 1844, he boarded the *Rio* and headed to New Providence to recover. During the voyage he made the acquaintance of two remarkable men, who would become lifelong friends. Edwin Charles Moseley was aboard the *Rio* with the printing press and equipment he had purchased in New York to start his newspaper, *The Nassau Guardian*. The Reverend Dr William Maclure was on his way to the pulpit of the St Andrews Presbyterian Kirk. Kirkwood reportedly contributed articles for the first issue of *The Nassau Guardian* and would worship at the Kirk for the rest of his life.[36]

In less than a decade, Kirkwood had built up the colony's most formidable practice. Income from his very busy private clinic was augmented by his responsibility for the recently formed Public Dispensary and the contract for the care of prisoners and the police. Kirkwood had the ear of the governor, as he was Gregory's personal physician. In addition, his influence was felt though his membership of the Legislative Council and his seat at the helm of the enterprise that controlled the colony's largest export, salt:[37] Kirkwood was chairman of the board of directors of the Inagua Salt Company.[38]

The messenger bypassed Cascadilla, and neither did he bother to see if Samuel Clutsam was on the island. He ran directly to the home of Dr Frederick Duncome and banged on the front door.

Duncome, 35, was born in Nassau, the second son of devout English parents. His elder brother, William Kelsall Duncome, was the first born Bahamian to be ordained an Anglican priest. Frederick studied medicine in Edinburgh and became the first native Bahamian to hold a medical diploma. He supplemented his practice income by serving as a medical officer to the local militia and doing weekly rounds at the New Providence Asylum, a duty that kept him in touch with the poor and destitute.[39] Medicine was Duncome's profession, but his passion was

Christian ministry. He was said to have been like the New Testament's Timothy, devout from youth and of a gentle and reserved disposition.[40] He was a vestryman of Christ Church and its representative at synod. He also happened to be the superintendent of Christ Church Sunday School.[41]

The young emissary, panting at Duncome's door, delivered his message. Without hesitation, the doctor grabbed his bag and followed the messenger out into the dark to Grants Town. The doctor found his patient gasping and unresponsive. The little girl had no fever or visible injury and there was nothing to suggest that she had a chronic disease. He inquired into what she had eaten during the day. When he learned that it had been bitter cassava for dinner, he knew in that instant the diagnosis.[42] For this condition, there was nothing that he could do. The child died that night from cyanide poisoning, a rare but well-recognised consequence of consuming cassava.[43]

The New Providence Asylum had begun in 1809 as a poor house on Shirley Street. By the 1850s, it had grown to encompass a collection of buildings that today we would call a nursing home.[44] There was no such thing as an emergency admission. To gain entry, one had to apply to one of its volunteer commissioners and provide a certificate of inability to pay, signed by a minister of religion. Its fifty-four residents, seventeen of whom the Blue Book summary reported belonged in a lunatic asylum, were given 'plain but wholesome' meals, which included a serving of turtle soup once a week.[45] It was the best-funded government health and welfare service, but not the only one. The government also maintained the Public Dispensary, a free ambulatory medical clinic.[46] The Dispensary was relatively new, created only in 1846, with the passage of 'An Act to mitigate the human suffering from poverty and disease'. It too required a formal application, supported by a note from a clergyman that certified poverty, to receive service.[47] Despite this hurdle, in 1851, over 1,200 residents sought care there. Most of them simply received medicine in accordance with a standard, pre-set formula, a device used well into the twentieth century.[48] Kirkwood, who was in charge of the institution, probably devoted no more than an hour or two to it each week.

The only other health service provided by the colony's government was the African Hospital. This institution, which gave Hospital Lane its name, was erected on West Hill Street, next door to the present-day National Art Gallery of The Bahamas. Its primary purpose was the care of African-born former slaves, and especially captives who had been rescued from slave ships by Britain's Royal Navy and released in New Providence. The brutality of the business had many of these individuals being sold into slavery seriously ill on arrival and their care became a state responsibility.

The first 450 of these liberated Africans, as they were known, were landed in 1811, four years after Great Britain outlawed the slave trade. In twenty-seven seizures up to 1860, more than 5,500 were resettled in The Bahamas.[49] Never having been enslaved and separated by a language barrier, this culturally distinctive group was cared for separately at the African Hospital.

The African Hospital was likely understaffed and of spartan accommodations, but the government had at least made some provision for liberated Africans. Its care of them had not always been praiseworthy. In 1832, Governor Carmichael-Smyth sent a group of 401 to Highbourne Cay while their legal status was debated in Sierra Leone. The several different ethnic groups were unable to communicate with each other. The authorities, expecting that they would grow their own food on the barren island, provided unfamiliar tools and seeds for cultivation. By the time word got back that the Africans were to be freed, 134 had died of starvation, exposure and disease.[50]

The approaching cholera epidemic would unite the colony's medical men to a single purpose, with the Board of Health the catalyst for their cooperation. The Board was formed by The Bahamas Parliament in 1850, two years after Great Britain had led the way;[51] Britain's Public Health Act of 1848, which created its General Board of Health, was crafted in response to the cholera epidemics erupting all over Europe.[52] Its purpose was to advise the government on public health matters and to enforce the Act through local Boards of Health in counties, towns and cities. These typically were comprised of a doctor, interested laymen and prominent citizens who were willing to serve. They hired sanitary inspectors, street sweepers and sewer repairmen. Britain's local boards also had the power to halt construction of a house or shut down a factory if it found that the building lacked a water closet.[53]

The Bahamas Board was superficially based on England's. However, its members were appointed by the governor rather than elected and it lacked the power to create contracts for public works – a power that it would temporarily acquire during the cholera epidemic.

Once the Board of Health was established, the Executive Council handed to it oversight of the New Providence Asylum (shared with the commissioners of the Asylum), the Dispensary and the African Hospital. Kirkwood and Chipman became founding members, joined by three of the colony's most prominent laymen: Felix MacCarthy, John F. Cook and John James Burnside.[54] MacCarthy had been the colony's police magistrate since 1846 and was responsible for maintaining law and order. Cook was the first provincial grand master for the Grand Masonic Lodge of Scotland in The Bahamas. Burnside (1782–1873) was the colony's surveyor-general and civil engineer.

The newly formed Board of Health admonished landowners in Nassau to keep their properties clean, upon pain of a fine of up to £10. It quoted Section IX of the Act.

> Section IX. And whereas, causes of sickness may arise from allowing weeds to grow, filth to accumulate or stagnant water to lie, or offensive substances to be brought within the several towns of the colony … or shall permit any description of filth or rubbish to accumulate therein, … [shall upon conviction be liable to a fine in a] sum not exceeding ten pounds.
> (Nassau, June 14, 1850)[55]

It reminded residents that it was now an offence to have outside toilets that were not a minimum of six feet deep. Weeds, rubbish, stagnant water and shallow toilets were together referred to as 'nuisances' – potential producers of the toxic miasma that led to cholera.

In much of New Providence, water was struck at a depth of four feet. The rule that outside toilets had to be at least six feet deep carried the risk that some residents could be targeted for selective harassment. However, the first public comment on the new Act was directed at the requirement that owners of property not permit any weeds to grow. A sharp-witted resident wrote the following.

> Upon what grounds the legislature came to the conclusion that allowing of weeds to grow may prove a cause of sickness, I am not informed. In this opinion, however I am not, in the face of all experience, and in defiance of the established facts of chemical science and vegetable physiology, prepared to concur. On the contrary, it is so thoroughly established that the living, growing vegetable organization is one of the grand purifiers of the atmosphere, and scavengers of creation, that it might seem superfluous to do more than state the fact. … living plants exercise a beneficial influence … the grand source of malaria is not from growing plants, but from dead and decaying vegetable and animal matters.[56]

I can imagine the writer smiling to himself as he continued to expound his logical argument.

> It is true that the law is intended to compel the removal of all rubbish 'within a reasonable time' but this reasonable time is not specified, nor the place where the accumulated debris of martyred vegetation, extensively cut down at this season in all its rank luxuriance, is to be deposited, to undergo that putrefactive decomposition, which, under the favourable influences of much moisture and a potent sun, is to generate its wholesale emanations of pestilential miasm. The 'reasonable time' should be *immediately*, for by the time the obnoxious shrubbery has *begun* to decay, or is dry enough to be burned, the mischief will have been done.

The writer's pushback had no noticeable effect, although it may have given pause to those who wrote the legislation – a reminder that rules made by the government needed to be well thought out.

One year after the Board of Health was formed, a census revealed the landscape of the population that it was formed to serve; the 1851 Census pegged the population at 27,219, an increase of 5,425 since Emancipation (see Appendix 13). It confirmed that residents of New Providence were concentrated in the Town District, but fully a third lived Over-the-Hill in Grants and Bain Town and in Fox Hill. There were only small settlements of liberated Africans and their descendants at Gambier and Adelaide.

The Census noted that an impressive 51 per cent of the population had been vaccinated against smallpox. Only a third could read and fewer could write.[57] An education, that key determinant of health and prosperity, was beyond the reach of the majority of the population. In theory, one was available at little or no cost. The government allocated £2,400 to fund twenty public schools and the Baptist Church, the Church of England and small private operators together added thirty-seven more.[58] Public schools had teachers that the government itself acknowledged were incompetent.[59] It treated them with contempt, paying a pittance of as little as £34 per annum (equivalent to less than $5,000 today).[60] In practice, only one in seven children was enrolled in any school and only half of those attended regularly.[61] Why would parents want to send their children to a lousy school when all hands were needed at the market and on the farm?

In the census year, Kirkwood, Chipman, MacCarthy and Cooke retired from the Board of Health. Burnside remained as the lone founding member and the governor appointed two new members in their stead: John Campbell Lees and James Black.[62]

Lees (1796–1873) was a veteran administrator who lived in an imposing residence called Hillside Manor on Cumberland Street, just steps from Government House.[63] He had not always enjoyed the favour of the commander-in-chief. In 1830, when he was an assistant judge, he had ignored Governor Carmichael-Smyth's prohibition on the corporal punishment of female slaves and authorised all of Lord Rolle's recaptured runaways to be flogged. Carmichael-Smyth promptly suspended him from the Executive Council and relieved him of his judicial appointment. Lees' show of defiance only increased his popularity among the local elite. At Emancipation, when Carmichael-Smyth was no longer governor, Lees was promoted to chief justice and now earned £850 annually.[64]

Black was a recent government hire, employed as the port health officer. Officially, he was the only person other than the harbour pilot who was permitted to board a vessel arriving from outside the colony. He inspected arriving passengers and crew and his permission was required to disembark. He enforced quarantine and kept a lookout for dangerous cargo – not arms, ammunition or explosives, but rotting produce and wet cotton, things believed to be carriers of disease.

Quarantine had long been the norm, but in the years preceding the cholera epidemic, enforcement had grown lax. The slackening was understandable, as yellow fever and smallpox had not been seen in the colony for years and cholera had never visited. One resident made it known that he was unhappy with the let-up. In May 1850, he complained to the editor of the *Bahama Herald* about a flagrant violation of the colony's quarantine laws that he had witnessed in the handling of the schooner *Iowa*. He fumed that the colony's quarantine procedures were nothing more than empty words on paper and that the quarantine officer's salary was a waste of money.[65]

By 1852, however, the climate had changed. The rising prevalence of smallpox and exploding epidemics of cholera in the region had motivated the colony to shore up its quarantine line of defence. In March, the House of Assembly passed new legislation 'to consolidate and amend the laws relating to Quarantine'. The amended Act was practically draconian. Previously, a ship was required to fly a yellow flag when someone aboard had yellow fever. The new Act bound the captain to declare whether anyone aboard had suffered any illness other than sea-sickness and, if so, to hoist a yellow flag. In a provision that reflected the level of the administration's fear, the Act gave the port health officer new sweeping powers while simultaneously quashing the debate about whether or not cholera was contagious. Black could impose quarantine even if everyone on board was in perfect health if he determined that 'any disease of a dangerous or contagious character, or of a *commonly supposed contagious* character has prevailed during the voyage'. The harbour pilot was required to present the captain of a vessel with a copy of the new Act when he boarded, to eliminate any pleas of ignorance.[66]

In May, Lees and Black were reappointed to the Board of Health, for terms that would run into the cholera epidemic.[67] However, at the time of their reappointment, the Board showed no interest in health measures that would benefit the general public. It never considered introducing maternal or childcare programmes. It employed no sanitary inspectors and it had no plans to improve the Dispensary or Asylum. Its first priority addressed the concerns of Nassau's merchants. The Board reconsidered its policy on wet cotton and decided to end the ban on its importation, ruling that wet cotton no longer had to be dumped in the ocean or buried, but could now be landed and dried on Hog Island.[68]

The governorship of John Gregory has been called 'undistinguished', but it spanned one of the most dramatic events in the archipelago's centuries of colonial rule.[69]

Gregory had been a bright lad, graduating in 1810 from The King's School with the distinction of being named Speech Day

Orator.[70] He began literature studies at the University of Edinburgh, but dropped out to enter the Foreign Service, starting as a paymaster's clerk in Malta and working his way up to become the colonial treasurer of Tasmania.[71] In 1848, at fifty-four years of age, Queen Victoria appointed him governor of The Bahamas. The greater part of his salary of £2,000 (approximately $260,000 today) was paid by the Colonial Office in London and he answered to its head, the secretary of state for the Colonies.[72] The Right Honourable Earl Grey (1802–1894) occupied that office as the cholera epidemic approached The Bahamas. In February 1852, Sir John Pakington (1799–1880) replaced him and ten months later, Henry Pelham-Clinton, the Duke of Newcastle (1811–1864) took over. They received informational mailings from Gregory, called despatches, which he signed, 'I have the honour to be Your Lordship's Most Obedient and Humble Servant.'

Gregory arrived in New Providence on Friday, March 2, 1849, alighting with his wife, two daughters, a son, his private secretary and three servants.[73] Acting Governor C. R. Nesbitt met the party at the dock and escorted them to Government House, where the members of the Executive Council were waiting. At 11 a.m. the following day, Chief Justice Lees swore him in.

The marginalised Black population were well aware that the authorities had minimal interest in their welfare. Still, they counted their blessings. In the colony they could find low-paid but seemingly stable employment as labourers in salt raking, pineapple farming, wrecking and sponging. The humiliating nightmare of slavery had ended and no epidemic diseases were present. Their Black brothers and sisters in The United States and

Cuba were still in bondage, living in communities that were battling outbreaks of smallpox, yellow fever and cholera. They welcomed the arrival of a new governor, holding a glimmer of hope that he might do a better job of looking out for their welfare.

The Venerable Archdeacon John Trew, mindful that his salary and those of his ten priests were paid by the government, composed the warmest of welcomes.[74]

> May the blessing of Almighty God abundantly rest upon your Excellency's administration, may the health of your lady and family be graciously preserved to you, and may that Gracious Providence which has brought you in safety to our shores direct that peace and happiness, truth and justice, religion and piety, may be established among us for all generations. We have the honour to be Sir, Your Excellency's obedient humble servants. Signed: J. M. Trew D.D., Archdeacon of The Bahamas. William Strachan, D.D., Rector of Christ Church. Joseph Maxwell, Rector of St Matthews. Henry MacDougall, A.M., Garrison Chaplain and Incumbent of St Mary's. Richard Chambers, A.B., Rector of St Ann and Minister of Carmichael, J. S. Higgs, Missionary and W. J. Woodcock, Curate of Grant's and Bain's Town.[75]

The new governor's first months were altogether pleasant. In October, the inhabitants of Pitts Cove, Eleuthera, flattered him with the petition to change the name of their area to Gregory Town. On November 10, he boarded the schooner *Violin*, accompanied by his aide-de-camp, J. B. Burnside, to begin a six-week tour of The Bahama Islands. In 1850, he oversaw the construction of St Ann's Parish Church 'in the African settlement of Sandilands'. He also saw the creation of Gregory's Arch, a tunnel next to Government House that burrowed through the limestone ridge, easing movement between Nassau and Bain and Grants Town, which the Blue Book called rural settlements 'chiefly populated by labourers of African birth or descent'.

In 1851, the governor was busy with the legislature. Twenty-one Acts were passed, including orders to build or to improve jails at Alice Town in Bimini, Harbour Island, Inagua, Eleuthera and Abaco.[76] A personal high point for the governor came on February 2, when Mrs Gregory bore a son in Government House.[77] Later in the month, he addressed the House of Assembly on the cholera pandemic, which the Colonial Office had been watching as it spread from Europe to the Americas. The Office knew that it presented a clear and present danger to The Bahamas and the governor briefed parliamentarians on what the Colonial Office had done in response. He painted the picture of a loving British Crown that was concerned for the welfare of its valued subjects.

> One of the most important subjects to which I referred is that of the public health, and with the view of showing how deep an interest her Majesty's government takes in all that concerns the West Indian colonies, and particularly the sanitary condition, I have a great satisfaction in equating your honorable house that I have this morning received from Earl Grey a despatch, announcing that three Medical

> Officers, highly distinguished for their professional attainments, have been sent out from England to afford the benefit of their advice and assistance to the local authorities, in adopting those precautionary measures the experience of Great Britain and Ireland has shewn to be most useful in checking the violence of Asiatic cholera.
>
> With your Honourable House, I sincerely trust, that it may please the Almighty to spare the Bahamas from this formidable scourge; but it will be satisfactory to know, that in the possible event of the calamity falling upon us, I should be enabled to summon one of these medical officers at once to our assistance, by communicating with Jamaica or Barbadoes.
>
> (John Gregory, Government House, Nassau, February 13, 1851)[78]

Exactly one year later, in February 1852, the governor was reminded of this resource when a letter arrived from Dr Hector Gavin, one of the West Indies medical inspectors. It informed of his presence in Trinidad and indicated that he would soon be available to the colony. Gavin had enclosed a copy of the report he had written on the cholera control measures he had implemented in Trinidad. He would be available, he said, for twelve months from April 12, at the daily rate of £3.3s (approximately $427 today).[79]

Gregory filed the communication away to concentrate on more pressing matters. On March 8, he told the House of Assembly of the Crown's intention to encourage free Black and mixed-race labourers in America to immigrate to The Bahamas to ease the labour shortage in salt production. On March 15, he swore in Stipendiary Magistrate Carleton. Newly arrived from London after a stint in Dominica, in a few short months, at the height of the cholera epidemic, he would be physically attacked for going where he was not welcome.

Gregory was somewhat distracted by preparations for his vacation. He had six months' leave coming up in April, which would cause him to miss the onset of the epidemic. However, he found time to report on the colony's finances and to seek London's confirmation of Dr Chipman's seat on the Legislative Council.[80]

In the days before his April 10 departure, longwinded letters of *bon voyage* to the governor appeared in the press. They praised his 'model of governance' and 'systematic administration'. Missives came from the Magistrates Chase, Inglis and Carleton and from the Speaker of the House of Assembly, who thanked the governor on behalf of the Members of Parliament for respecting their privileges as 'representatives of the people'. A letter from Chief Justice Lees lauded the governor on behalf of the Legislative Council. Another, signed by 110 distinguished residents who made the preposterous claim of being 'humble inhabitants of the colony', gushed, 'we beg to express our sincere wish that He who governs the winds and seas may protect you and your family to your native country and we beg to assure you, that we will be happy to hail your return among us'.[81]

Colonial Secretary Nesbitt was one of the 110 signatories. He had come to Nassau from England as a child in 1815, when his father was the colony's colonial secretary. He worked his way up the administration and, upon his father's demise in 1838, was officially appointed to the position.[82] Nesbitt would go down as the most powerful civil servant in the history of the colony. During the cholera epidemic, the power of his pen would be felt by everyone.

Other names appended to the governor's *bon voyage* included Provost Marshal Munnings, along with the clergy, merchants, lawyers and doctors. Stephen Dillet and John Minns, the only Black Members of Parliament, also signed. Captain John Hall, who would transport the governor to Philadelphia aboard the *Victoria*, signed, as did Captain Evans. Their over-the-top flattery bore genuine affection. Many of them would have remembered the stormy relationship they had suffered with Governor Carmichael-Smyth only too well. He had bulldozed his opposition, while Gregory by comparison was a consensus-builder and open to consultation.

No actual humble inhabitants signed the published letter of farewell or had the audacity to write independently. They knew that they were insignificant and invisible as far as the administration was concerned. Perhaps they would be noticed when the governor returned?

❦ ❦ ❦

Colonial Secretary Nesbitt became acting governor – and not for the first time – while Gregory was away. He promoted Magistrate William Robert Inglis, a resident of Green Turtle Cay, to the post of acting colonial secretary.

The Board of Health presently had little on its plate. Administration of the New Providence Asylum fell under the responsibility of a separate group of commissioners. The African Hospital was hardly taxing and no improvement initiatives were afoot. In June, Nesbitt gave Lees additional responsibilities; he and Kirkwood were appointed to the colony's first Board of Works.[83]

This Board was immediately busy on an area east of the town of Nassau, which from Dowdeswell Street to the Eastern Parade was known as the Swamp Grounds. A concerted effort to fill it in and to organise drainage had started earlier. In 1835, Lieutenant Governor William Colebrooke had earned credit for the 'enlightened exertions' that completed the bulk of the work. However, the job was still ongoing in 1851, with the focus on eliminating the foul odours from stagnant pools. The colonial secretary reported with satisfaction that the drains had been cleared of mud and 'faced and soled with stone under the supervision of the civil engineer'.[84]

Medicine is replete with examples like this one, where mistaken observations lead to measures that ultimately prove beneficial for the wrong reasons. The elimination of the swamplands next to the town, aimed at the suppression of foul odours, disrupted mosquito breeding grounds, helping to keep malaria and yellow fever out of New Providence. The measures could not prevent contamination of the water table, though, which is what happened when a sailor brought in cholera and touched off an epidemic.

# 2

## Cholera in the Region

Jean Salgadeau Pelette, 38, was placid when he was taking his medication. Well-known to the people of Mirebalais, he generally kept to himself. However, when off his medication, he could be found wandering about the town, dirty, naked and conversing with invisible companions.

Pelette may have been too ill to work, but he was neither homeless nor destitute. He came from a prominent family and they took the best care of him that he would allow. He had his own room, a place behind a shop off the town square. Most mornings, he ambled down the hill from his place to the Latem River to bathe and drink. This tributary to Haiti's mighty Artibonite River ran right through the town and numerous townsfolk used it to drink, to clean up before school and to do laundry.

On January 12, 2010, a 7.0-magnitude earthquake centred fifty miles from Mirebalais shook Port-au-Prince. It killed almost 100,000 people outright, injured another 300,000 and rendered over a million suddenly homeless. The earthquake also disrupted

Haiti's already inadequate water and sewerage system, providing fertile ground for a secondary disaster from disease caused by contaminated water.

Mirebalais swelled with displaced relatives who had somewhere to go other than the vast refugee camps. United Nations soldiers and relief workers from multiple countries came to render aid. Ten months after the earthquake, a detachment from Nepal set up camp two miles upstream from Mirebalais and the soldiers gave little thought to discharging their waste into the river. By then, the townsfolk had returned to their morning routine at the Latem. On the afternoon of October 16, Pelette was found sprawled on the riverbank, groaning, soiled in his own excrement and too weak to move. He was carried to his room, where Malherbe, his brother and a future president of the local Rotary Club, cleaned him off and put him to bed. No one realised the mortal danger at hand and when Malherbe checked back at 4 p.m., his brother was dead from cholera.

The disease spread from Mirebalais throughout the country, following the course of the river. Pelette was tagged as Haiti's first case – its Patient Zero.[85] All evidence pointed to the Nepalese camp as the disease's origin, but only in September 2016 did the UN secretary-general admit the organisation's culpability.[86]

The outbreak of cholera in Haiti sent shockwaves to Bahamas public health officials. They quickly produced posters with information on cholera prevention and placed them in public buildings and at schools. A spotter was placed at the airport to eyeball arriving passengers and healthcare providers were updated. One year into the epidemic in Haiti, a Royal Bahamas Defence Force vessel intercepted a Haitian sloop loaded with would-be undocumented immigrants. One of them was suffering with severe watery diarrhoea and subsequent tests confirmed that he was suffering from cholera.

While the Ministry had previously been criticised for its slow-as-molasses response to an earlier dengue epidemic, on this occasion officials moved with blazing speed. On October 21, by the time of the minister of health's announcement that cholera had been diagnosed in a would-be immigrant, the detainee had already been treated and repatriated, along with all forty-seven of his compatriots. In addition, the entire population of the Carmichael Road Detention Centre had been transferred to the Department of Corrections in Fox Hill to allow the Centre to be disinfected.

A local outbreak was averted, but exactly one year later, in October 2012, a twenty-three-year-old who was pregnant with a near-term baby turned up at the emergency room of the Princess Margaret. The woman, who had been doing well until only a few hours earlier, arrived in a state of collapse. She had severe diarrhoea, with watery stool that looked like rice water. She went into premature labour and miscarried, and she too nearly died. Tests proved that her disease was cholera. Stunned officials determined that the lady had not been outside of The Bahamas, yet, despite their best detective efforts, the local source of her disease remained a mystery.[87]

Cholera has always killed in the manner that it cut down Pelette in Mirebalais. Its hallmark is watery diarrhoea, with effluent that looks like rice water. Sunken eyes, leathery skin and painful leg cramps from severe dehydration quickly appear. There is no fever, bloody stool or mental confusion, as happens in typhoid. In fact, cholera victims are often lucid and communicative right up until the moment that they suddenly die.

The disease was to the Victorian era what the plague had been in Europe five centuries earlier: a reaper of families and a destroyer of towns. Tuberculosis may have killed more people in total, but it did so slowly as it haunted areas for generations. Sufferers could live for years with intermittent night fevers, ghastly weight loss and coughing up blood.[88] Cholera, by contrast, arrived like a storm, caused a massacre and then disappeared for decades. Few towns had the opportunity to become familiar with the disease, as would have been the case with tuberculosis.

Cholera was believed to be caused by an inhaled poison called a miasma, produced by rotting matter in soil and which floated into the air. Yellow fever and malaria (from Italian *mala aria*, literally 'bad air') were thought to be of similar origin. The name cholera comes from the Greek *kholéra,* meaning 'a flow of bile'. It was actually considered to be a collection of diseases, among which watery diarrhoea just happened to be a common symptom. In addition to subdividing this one disease, doctors confused any number of other causes of diarrhoea with cholera.

Thomas Sydenham (1624–1689), a great English physician, spelled out the difference between what was called common cholera, or *cholera morbus*, and dysentery. Persons with the latter illness saw blood in the stool and had *tenesmus* (a painful urge to defecate).[89] Sydenham was handy with the rough remedies of the day, but he was especially appreciated for the gentle therapies that he favoured. For cholera morbus and dysentery he prescribed *accubitus* (the touch of a warm body).

> In May 1662, when called to see a Mrs. Change, very ill of a cholera morbus, he got her husband to lie naked close to her back and her son, aged 12, against her belly. Their natural heat soon resuscitated the patient. He treated a woman for dysentery by causing her son, a plump, hot lad of thirteen years of age, and her nurse's son of six or seven years, to go to bed to her naked and to lie the one close to her belly, the other close to her back, which they did, and so long as they continued with her she had no stools; but the boys rising at any time the looseness would immediately return. I commanded that she should persist in her course till her cure should be complete (the boys relieving one another by turns in the daytime) and so she fully recovered.[90]

Nineteenth-century physicians, including those in The Bahamas, believed that cholera was caused by a poisonous miasma which came from rotting garbage and damp soil and was carried in the air. It targeted the poor, they said, because they lived in cramped quarters, lacked faith in God, abused alcohol, were immoral and were susceptible to panic. Politicians and the clergy called it a divine punishment sent to bring people closer to God. They advocated fasting and prayer for protection and when an epidemic ended, its termination was attributed to the success of prayer. Any mild diarrhoea might be a 'promontory symptom' that could become 'near cholera' if it persisted. Doctors tried to convince the public that proper treatment of the promontory symptom – meaning their prescriptions alone – could prevent progression to the feared and often-fatal 'variety'. That variety was the one that came from Asia, called *cholera asiatica* or 'The Cholera'.[91] Even the most optimistic physician tempered his hyperbole of the dependability of his medicines when faced with a patient in the grip of full-blown cholera asiatica.

In 1855, John Snow published his classic work *On the Mode of Communication of Cholera.*[92] In it, he detailed how he had mapped cases in the Soho district of London, connecting them with contaminated water supplies. After he had convinced the city commissioners to remove the pump handle from the public pump on Broad Street, cholera deaths abruptly stopped. Snow's detractors remained unconvinced and argued that the drop in cases merely reflected the natural tendency of an epidemic to end on its own. They also pointed to the fact that an unknown number of residents had fled to the countryside with the onslaught of the epidemic. Their arguments were sufficiently convincing to muddy the water and the miasma theory not only persisted but was aggressively defended by influential experts. The anti-contagionists, as they were known, were championed by Edwin Chadwick (1800–1890) in London and by Max von Pettenkofer (1818–1901), a professor of medical chemistry in Munich.

Nations continued to depend on quarantine to keep out what was believed to be an airborne disease. Quarantine, from the Italian *quaranta*, meaning 'forty', was introduced in Europe in the 1300s to keep the plague epidemic at bay.[93] It entailed a forty-day period of enforced separation of persons, animals and goods, and for the plague, to some degree, it worked. The emergence of cholera pandemics reactivated plague-era strategies. New 'pest houses' were built for the isolation of the sick and nations revived quarantine regulations. The rules varied from place to place and the difficulty of enforcing the hodge-podge of different systems at each port became a major drag on trade. In addition, there was lots of evidence to show that quarantine was not actually keeping cholera at bay, despite it having the strong support of a panicked citizenry.

A series of International Sanitary Conferences was convened to discuss cholera and to design uniform regulations on quarantine, with Pettenkofer a delegate at both the second, in 1859, and the third, in 1866, where Snow's findings were first ignored and then derided.[94] Finally, in 1883, Robert Koch rediscovered and isolated the *Vibrios* first seen by Filippo Pacini in 1854, and their existence was widely accepted and the miasma dogma discredited. William Osler's *The Principles and Practice of Medicine*, the physicians' bible at the turn of the twentieth century, was updated to plainly state that cholera was caused by the consumption of food or water contaminated by faeces. However, the textbook acknowledged the persistence of a stubborn fringe that opposed 'the drinking water theory'.

Today, we know more: that the cholera *Vibrio* thrives in brackish water, that the organisms attach to and infect the intestinal lining of humans, and that they produce a toxin called choleragin, or CTX. It is this toxin which makes cholera such a distinctive and deadly disease. CTX poisons specific proteins in the cells of the intestine, and can cause a life-threatening hyperactivation of secretory channels with the active pumping of fluid from the circulation into the intestinal tract. This actually only happens in a minority of those who encounter the bacteria.

Most persons who become infected do not become ill, but simply carry and excrete the *Vibrios,* with some 10 per cent doing so for three weeks or more. A small minority can become long-term carriers.[95]

While the correct knowledge of how to prevent cholera came in the second half of the nineteenth century, effective treatment lagged behind. *The Merck Manual*, which grew from a useful physician's pocket reference into the world's best-selling medical textbook, listed no fewer than sixty treatments for cholera in its 1899 first edition. They included arsenic, morphine, cannabis, chloral hydrate and chloroform. Thankfully, turpentine, today used as a paint solvent, had fallen away as a remedy and was included only as an antiseptic for application to cancerous growths.[96]

Intravenous therapy was the first lifesaving measure developed, but it has the major drawback that it requires advanced training, technical equipment and sterile supplies. These things have traditionally been scarce or unavailable where cholera is common. Oral rehydration therapy was introduced in the 1960s after decades of research into the electrolyte transport mechanisms in the intestine.[97] This therapy cut the death rate for cholera from 40–50 per cent down to 1 per cent, and in 1978 the World Health Organization (WHO) finally adopted it as the treatment of choice for cholera – and now for all infectious diarrhoea.

The cradle of the disease has always been the Ganges Delta of India and Bangladesh. In the past two centuries, it has burst out to cause worldwide pandemics seven times. In 1817, it spread over six years from Calcutta to several countries in Asia, losing steam after reaching the Philippines. Ten years later, epidemics spread far beyond Asia, to Great Britain and across the Atlantic to Canada and the United States.[98] In 1833, cholera reached Cuba, with the city of Havana losing 8,253 from a population of 65,000. The rest of the Caribbean remained unscathed.[99] The third pandemic, the one that would ravage the West Indies and come to The Bahama Islands, was touched off in 1839 by British troops stationed in India. They carried the disease into Afghanistan and the following year it appeared in China. In 1848, it reached the seething and squalid cities of the Old World. In July, the disease erupted in Berlin; in October, it was in London and Edinburgh. In December, the disease reached Belfast.[100] Across the Atlantic, the European spread of cholera was watched with alarm. The ocean was no longer the foreboding barrier that it had been a decade earlier. Transporting immigrants to America had become a routine and profitable business.

In 1848, New York was America's largest, most important and undeniably filthiest city. There was no effective system of garbage collection. The wild hogs, goats and dogs that roamed the streets were its most efficient refuse disposal agents. On December 2, 1848, after twenty-two days at sea, the packet ship *New York* reached Staten Island with a new batch of emigrants. She had departed from Havre-de-Grâce, France with over 300 of them stuffed below in steerage. When she dropped anchor, seven lay dead and numerous others had the unmistakable symptoms of cholera.

Authorities quickly converted the customs warehouses on Staten Island into a makeshift hospital for the immigrants. Another thirty died there before the year was out, but half of those quarantined on the island climbed the fence, hopped into small boats and dispersed into the city. Cholera began to appear in New York City within a week and, in May 1849, after a winter hibernation, a full-blown epidemic erupted. Bodies piled up faster than they could be carted away and corpses lay on the streets for days before being taken to Randall's Island to be buried in shallow graves. Within two months, over 5,000 residents had died and business came to a virtual standstill.[101]

The disease was spread southwards along trade routes and westwards by gold-seekers. News of it in New Orleans led a letter-writer in The Bahamas to remark on the precarious position of the colony. Christianus wrote the following to the editor of the *Bahama Herald.*

> Cholera has been raging within a few days sail of us for months, yet we have, through the mercy of God, been hitherto spared. Can we honestly say that such immunity is owing to any superior claims on our part? Assuredly not. 'But to the Lord our God belong mercies and forgiveness, though we have rebelled against Him. He has not dealt with us after our sins, nor rewarded us after our iniquities.' May He still graciously avert what may yet come upon us, and make us 'to show forth our gratitude not only with our lips but in our lives,' for the abundant mercy He has hitherto shewn us![102]

Everywhere, cholera's victims were mainly poor, although the high and mighty were also cut down. In June 1849, it killed former US President James Polk and then his successor, President Zachary

Taylor, shortly after he had championed a day of fasting and prayer to ward off the epidemic.[103]

In Cuba, authorities imposed a strict quarantine on vessels from the United States, but in March 1850, the disease found an opening and for a second time sneaked into Havana. As the year drew to a close and the pace of new cases appeared to be slackening, officials pronounced the epidemic to be over, while hiding the fact that over 6,000 residents had lost their lives to the disease. Ultimately, a total of 17,144 deaths were counted in the official toll. The statistics were confounded with an outbreak of a smallpox, but Kiple estimated that Cuba lost between 8 and 10 per cent of its slave population, or 26,000–34,000 lives, during the epidemic of the 1850s.[104]

Seven months after cholera had appeared in Cuba, the disease attacked Jamaica.

* * *

Port Royal, the scene of the first case of cholera in Jamaica, had once been a rich and lawless pirate haven. In the middle of the nineteenth century, it had fallen to become a shabby community of boatmen, fishermen and washerwomen. The admiral of the West India regiment stationed on the island had predicted that, should it ever be introduced there, cholera would decimate the grimy town.

It did, beginning with Nancy Johnston, a fifty-year-old Black woman who shared a beachfront shack with several housemates in the part of the town where residents went to relieve themselves and to empty their waste buckets. On the night of October 6,

1850, Nancy developed severe diarrhoea, which came on so suddenly it was described as a seizure, and she died the following afternoon. By the end of the week, thirty or more of her Port Royal neighbours were dead from cholera. It claimed over 200 of the town's 1,000 residents, including Nancy's housemates. None of the victims came from the comfortable minority, the 'well housed and the well fed'.[105]

On October 8, a fisherman named Phipps became the first victim in Kingston. According to Milroy's report on the epidemic, he lived 'in one of the filthy negro yards' at the upper end of Oxford Street. As was typical of the disease, he developed diarrhoea and belly pain and died within hours. His neighbour was next, a young girl who lived across the street, and then someone who lived near the Spanish Town Road. Bodies piled up as a full-blown epidemic tore through the communities and then spread across the island faster than the news. Nurse Mary Seacole, a Kingston innkeeper, became a cholera treatment expert by watching 'a Dr B, – who was then lodging in my house'. Her confidence, combined with her newfound skill, would be put to good use later, when she would travel to South America and to Crimea. Like her contemporary Florence Nightingale, she was revered, and, for a time after the publication of her 1857 memoir, almost as famous.[106]

The governor of Jamaica's initial report to Earl Grey on the epidemic was sent that October. London's halls of power were quickly inundated with cries for help from bankers, merchants and brokers in London – men who did business in Jamaica.[107] In December, Jamaica's legislature even drew up a petition asking Her Majesty to send all liberated Africans to the island to make up the labour shortage caused by the cholera epidemic. To address the shortage of health professionals, businessmen called on the British government to mount a large-scale medical mission, with boatloads of doctors and medical supplies. In the wake of Emancipation, in what has been described as Jamaica's first brain-drain, there had been an exodus of doctors from the colony, with medical practitioners in short supply even before the cholera epidemic made the shortage acute.[108]

Without waiting for a government mission, John Parkin (1801–1888), a physician with a thriving mental health practice in Piccadilly who dabbled as an expert in diseases of the potato, took it upon himself to travel to Kingston to help.[109] He was familiar with the system of house-to-house visitation that the General Board of Health recommended to discover and treat early cases. He landed in Jamaica on December 26, 1850, and it did not take him long to conclude that on the island, house-to-house visitation was both impractical and futile.[110] For one thing, there were not enough trained personnel to attend to the sick, much less to visit apparently healthy homes. For another, he found that in numerous instances he visited homes in the morning, where he met vigorous young individuals, only to discover when he returned in the evening that someone had died from cholera during the day and had already been buried.[111]

The large-scale medical mission called for never materialised. London's General Board of Health convinced the Secretary of State that this would be a futile exercise, since the epidemic might be over before such a mission could be assembled and transported. The Board conceived of a completely different taskforce, one comprised of specialists in public health who would not get their hands dirty treating cholera cases, but who would rather be advisors to the local authorities on preventative measures. They would be called West Indies medical inspectors.[112]

Three London-based physicians with impressive public health credentials were identified by the Board: Gavin Milroy, Hector Gavin and a Dr Laidlaw. On January 1, 1851, Earl Grey appointed each to the newly created office of 'Medical Inspector to the West Indies' for a one-year term at a salary of £1,500 plus expenses. Each was intimately familiar with the two main cholera-combatting strategies that the General Board of Health promoted: early diagnosis and treatment by house-to-house visits and the clean-up of environmental waste to eliminate the noxious poisons produced by rotting matter in soil.

The General Board of Health had not needed to look far for its appointees. Gavin Milroy (1805–1886), the first of them, was already employed as an inspector with the London Board. He had obtained his medical education in his native city of Edinburgh, and in the 1840s had gained experience in the Caribbean as a physician aboard the government Packet Service. His experiences had made him no fan of quarantine. His 1846 publication *On Plague and Quarantine* was the first of multiple assaults he made on the quarantine regulations. In it, he wrote: 'The absurdly foolish and most ridiculous principles which [they] embody, the vexatious and oppressive restriction which they impose, their wretchedness and suffering which they almost necessarily give rise to, and the great increase to mortality which, we have reason to believe, they often occasion, are surely sufficient grounds for the scrutinizing investigation that is so generally demanded.'[113] In 1850, his public health profile was enlarged when he became a founding member of the London Epidemiological Society.[114]

Laidlaw, the second appointee, appeared and faded with little recorded about him. I could discover only that he had been physician to the consulate at Alexandria, that he had gained some experience in the treatment of cholera in tropical climates and that at some point he had written a 'valuable paper' on the plague.[115]

Hector Gavin (1815–1855) was the most colourful of the West Indies inspectors and the one who wound up in The Bahamas. He too was a native of Edinburgh, the son of an engraver and a whiz-kid in his youth. At sixteen years of age, he was an apprentice with the Royal College of Surgeons of Edinburgh. At nineteen, he won the College's Gold Medal for Botany and at age twenty, he wrote an intellectually precocious and prize-winning paper titled 'On Feigned and Factitious Diseases Chiefly of Soldiers and Seamen, On the Means Used to Simulate or Produce them and on the Best Modes of Discovering Impostors'.[116] At twenty-one, he was a qualified and licensed physician. He started a private practice in London and lectured in forensic medicine at the Charing Cross Hospital. Gavin supplemented his income as a visitor to the London Orphan Asylum and to the British Penitent Female Refuge. In 1847, he signalled his passion for public health with the publication of a number of papers and the release of his first book, *The Unhealthiness of London*. He also took duties at a workhouse in the district of Bethnal Green, where he did the work that led to his best-known publication, *Sanitary Ramblings*. That same year, 1848, he was elevated to the Fellowship of the Royal College of Surgeons of Edinburgh and he became secretary to the newly formed body, which was now employing him to go to the West Indies.

*Sanitary Ramblings* revealed Gavin's prodigious energy as he mapped out, street by street, the layout and condition of the Parish of Bethnal Green. It concluded with a scathing indictment of the district's authorities: 'The conclusion at which we must necessarily arrive, when the preceding facts have been duly weighed, is, that if the inhabitants of Bethnal-Green must wait till those sanitary improvements which are so urgently required for their physical and moral welfare, shall be executed by their own authority; centuries, and even ages may pass away with but little change from the present state of things.' He called the authorities incompetent and worse.

> The authorities are not only utterly incapable of designing, superintending, or executing great public works, but they cannot be led to conceive their necessity. No loud demand has ever been made by them for increased sewage, or appeal to their constituents for support to obtain it. No works of drainage, whether in connection with the sewers which already exist, or to improve the present miserable condition of house and street drainage, have been executed by them. No supplies of water have been sought to cleanse their drains, or streets; no means but in the most imperfect character have been adopted to remove refuse from the streets; and the contracts to remove refuse from the houses, whether of rich or poor, but especially from the houses of the poor, have been scandalously neglected; and the short-coming of the contractors most unaccountably glossed over.

He poked the district commissioners right in the eye in his conclusion.

> It is presumed that the most solid reason for the wretched condition of the great majority of the houses of the poor, and for the total absence of any attempts at improvement, consists in the fact that the Commissioners and guardians are themselves the chief proprietors of the dwellings of the poor, and that as they, in general pay the rates themselves, and have already exacted for their tenements the highest attainable rents, any, even the slightest increase, of rates would only be an increase of their own expenditure. Under such circumstances, but the narrow and limited views entertained by such parties, to expect permanent and effectual improvements at the most limited present expenditure appears perfectly fallacious.[117]

The book came back to bite him when he applied for the position of medical officer of health for the City of London. In public health credentials, he was the strongest of the twenty-two candidates and he made the final cut, but the city commissioners had read his book. They grilled him over his apparent disdain of the authorities and specifically about the concluding paragraph of his *Sanitary Ramblings*.[118] He pled that his writings referred only to the Bethnal Green district and not to the whole London metropolis, but to no avail.[119] The disappointment left him available to accept the invitation to become a West Indies medical inspector. The Board's familiarity with him seems to have overriden any concerns they may have held over whether a man with such a stunning lack of diplomacy was the best candidate to represent the British government overseas.

Laidlaw and Hector Gavin were directed to Barbados, selected due to the regional military command's headquarters there. The Colonial Office believed that interaction with the military surgeons would be a good starting point for doctors about to wage a medical war. The Office gave the pair latitude to change their destination if they found upon their arrival at the transfer hub of St Thomas, which is today one of the US Virgin Islands, that their services were more urgently wanted elsewhere. Their instructions were that, 'On reaching each colony which you may visit, you will in the first instance report yourself to the Governor or Lieutenant Governor and you will then, after receiving his general instructions, proceed to the islands and examine the state of the preparations made for meeting the epidemic.'[120] Gavin and Laidlaw made it safely to Barbados. Hector shifted his headquarters to Port of Spain, Trinidad after a few weeks, and from there he launched excursions to Tobago, Grenada and St Vincent. Laidlaw fell seriously ill and returned to London, where he died a few months later. In British Guiana, Gavin contracted yellow fever, which nearly killed him. He convalesced at his new headquarters in Port of Spain.[121]

Gavin Milroy was sent to the hotspot, Jamaica. He arrived there on January 28, 1851. By then, thousands had died and all business, except that of coffinmaking and gravedigging, had stopped. Although he tried to maintain a clinical distance, Milroy's reporting betrayed his shock at the depth of poverty he encountered and at the ravages of cholera, which in the end left

40,000 persons dead.[122] The sheer number of corpses in every town hit overwhelmed any semblance of orderly burial. Some were left to be picked to pieces by vultures and hogs. Many more went into mass graves. A few – maybe more – were buried alive.

The belief that cholera corpses were super-spreaders, especially immediately after death, caused persons who were critically ill to be abandoned. This happened everywhere, including in The Bahamas. In Jamaica, people burned huts to the ground with bodies inside rather than risking infection by approaching a corpse. Families discarded the useless medicines provided by authorities and began to dig a grave the moment a relative developed cholera symptoms. Some were known to have a rope placed around their neck so that, without anyone having to get too close, they could be dragged to the grave the moment they breathed their last. Actual confirmation of death was very much an inexact science in the 1850s, and the not-quite-dead were buried often enough that Jamaica's Central Board of Health issued a public scolding in 1854.

> There is one point regarding the contagious or infectious property of the disease, which the Central Board of Health would particularly allude to. It is the supposed increase of infection about the dead body. The members of the board would express their conviction, that such is not the case. If the dead body is at all infectious, it is unphilosophical and absurd to suppose that it can be more so, *coeteris paribus*, than the living body, and they maintain that such theory has been proved experimentally to be quite unfounded. The

> Central Board are persuaded, that where there is cleanliness and free ventilation, there is nothing to be dreaded from a cholera corpse above any other corpse. The contrary opinion led during the last epidemic to some of the most horrid and inhumane acts on the part of friends and nearest relatives, and, it is to be feared, was in several instances the cause of persons being interred alive.[123]

Milroy suggested that the burying alive of victims was a manifestation of the backwardness and depravity of Black people. He was spouting unadulterated ignorance and prejudice. Accidental live burial was an ancient hazard and it remains a risk to the present day.[124] Long before the cholera epidemic, in Germany and France, researchers had carefully documented dozens of instances.[125] The artist Antoine Joseph Weirtz witnessed it first-hand during a cholera epidemic in Naples, a trauma that inspired his famous painting *The Premature Burial.*[126]

Racism was not merely evident in Milroy's assessment of the behaviour of Black residents about the island. It was also evident in his conduct towards the prisoners housed at the General Penitentiary in Kingston. Medical research on Black prisoners has a long and sad history.[127] During the colonial era, physicians took advantage of the enslaved and imprisoned to study disease. The knowledge gained and shared by doctors made and enlarged their careers.[128] Milroy would not pass up this opportunity. He visited the Penitentiary, where 508 inmates were housed, only seven of whom were White. On October 13, a group of 100 prisoners were taken out to clean the streets. A gang of them worked near the home of fisherman

Phipps. Milroy anticipated an outbreak among the inmates and he set out to study how long the disease took to kill. On October 15, when the first inmate developed symptoms, Milroy (or a flunky) marked the time when he fell ill and then counted the hours until he died. The indifferent investigator watched 128 prisoners die, with no mention of any treatment attempted. Milroy included the data obtained as a table in his 154-page report to London.

Milroy saw that prisoners' drinking water came from wells as shallow as one foot in depth. The undoubtedly contaminated water proved no impediment to Milroy finding the prisoners themselves partly to blame for their disease: 'It does not belong to the present narrative to do more than merely allude, in passing, to the revolting disclosures of horrible vice among the prisoners made before a committee in 1850. Moral and physical pollution go hand in hand.' [129]

| No. of inmates | Duration from onset to death |
|---|---|
| 4 | 6 hours |
| 41 | 6–12 hours |
| 28 | 12–18 hours |
| 15 | 18–24 hours |
| 22 | 1–2 days |
| 6 | 2–3 days |
| 6 | 4–5 days |
| 5 | 7–9 days |
| 1 | 9–10 days |
| **Total 128** | |

Table 1. Duration of cholera attacks in the Kingston Penitentiary, October 15 through November 20, 1850. [130]

Milroy also blamed Black people, in part, for the fact that some doctors had left practice or gone broke. They would not employ a doctor, he said, even when they could afford one. Still, he appealed to the Colonial Office to help the poor and barely civilised former slaves because it was Britain's Act of Emancipation that had caused the problem. The Act was the instrument:

by which a semi-barbarous people were hastily released from care and protection as well as from the oppression and ignominy of servitude, measures were not devised or precautions taken to provide for the change which would inevitably ensure in the condition of the people. One of the most disastrous of the results as unquestionably been the progressively diminishing supply of medical assistance, until, as of recent years, many large portions of the country have been left nearly bare in this respect.[131]

The well-travelled medical inspector was as wedded to the fallacy of White racial superiority as any lowly colonial clerk. At least he meant well, and he departed Jamaica after eight months, annoyed at the governor's foot-dragging over the enactment of his suggested improvements to the island's public health legislation.

Milroy's term was cut short because he was wanted as a delegate to the Sanitary Conference in France. The Conference came out of an initiative to seek an agreed international protocol on quarantine and to rationalise the hodgepodge of port regulations.[132] In July of 1851, Paris hosted the first of several of these conferences. Delegations comprised of a physician and a diplomat and all of the great European powers were represented. Somehow, Milroy's preparation to represent Britain neglected to resolve the discrepancy between his personal opposition to quarantine and his government's practice of enforcing it. In the end, the conference voted to implement a period of fifteen days for ships coming from a port with yellow fever and five days for those from a cholera port. Milroy's vocal opposition to quarantine must have been a little awkward for Britain, because it remained official government policy and it was enforced in its West Indies colonies.[133 134]

❦ ❦ ❦

By the end of 1851, Hector Gavin was the only one of the three West Indies medical inspectors contracted for a year-long tour of duty who was still on the job. He remained busy in Trinidad and, certain that there would be more for him to do in the region, applied for a twelve-month extension of his commission. It was granted, on the condition that each territory he visited pay half his remuneration of £3.3s a day.

# 3

# Hall Lane

In the 1850s, senior government officials, merchants and professionals in The Bahamas inhabited a charmed plateau. This clique prospered, while the mass of uneducated former slaves suffered under a regime of near-slave wages. White residents in the middle of the social pyramid had no easy road. Farming, wrecking, sponging and supervising salt-rakers was strenuous work. A few White men who were outside of the elite but who possessed special skills did better than their peers. One of those was Samuel Evans.[135]

Evans was in high demand as one of the colony's most capable boat captains. In an age when all people and goods were transported by sea, he was busy and well paid. In May 1852, he captained the *Elector* on a sponging trip to Abaco.[136] In June, he took the *Reform* to Turks Island and back, and in July, he led the *Elizabeth* out on a wrecking mission.[137]

The *Reform* was a new thirty-seven-ton schooner, first registered on October 2, 1850.[138] Her owners had her designed for speed, to facilitate their business of conveying passengers and cargo throughout the Caribbean and to the United States. In August 1852, they needed a shipment of Eleuthera pineapples delivered to New York and Evans was entrusted with this mission.

The trip to New York was uneventful but the sailors had a dreadful stay. Cholera was raging in the city and all of the men came down with some stomach upset. They may have had mild attacks of cholera, but one sailor became seriously ill and died from the disease. On September 8, the *Reform* returned to Nassau a man short, loaded with a cargo of flour, meal, potatoes and onions.[139] The Nassau port health officer found no evidence of disease and permitted the crew to land.[140] Evans made himself comfortable at lodgings near the Eastern Parade, while the ship, at anchor nearby, was cleaned and fumigated.

Opposite the Eastern Parade lived Ann Hall. She was sixty and a widow, still strong and charming. Ann loved men of the sea. Her late husband, Captain John Hall, was a master mariner who, like most successful White men of his day, had been a slaveowner. In 1824, Ann had become Captain Hall's second wife at St Matthew's Church and they lived nearby.[141] The street where the couple made their home bore his name, Hall Lane.[142] Their only son, John Robert Hall, followed his father into the maritime profession.

Harbour Island was a hub of boatbuilding and it was where John Robert Hall found and married Frances Mary (nee Sweeting). In 1852, John Robert was twenty-seven years old, with a family of his own and a position as commander of the *Victoria.* This passenger vessel was owned by a pair of Philadelphia businessmen and Hall sailed her regularly between Nassau and the city of love.[143] She carried up to twenty passengers, many of whom were only in transit through the colony as immigrants to America.[144] Hall set out on his third or fourth trip to Philadelphia for the year in the same month as Evans set out for New York with pineapples. His family was expecting him back any day, and when Ann got word that Evans was in town, she paid him a visit.[145]

The record states that Ann went to obtain news about her son; that there may have been additional motivations for the visit would be pure speculation. There is no denying that Evans would have been the person to ask for intelligence on the progress and whereabouts of the *Victoria.* How long she stayed is not known. She was probably offered a cool drink as she stepped out of the heat, and perhaps she shared a fruit or some treat brought back from New York. All we know for certain is that within a day or two of her visit, she suddenly developed severe diarrhoea. She had only been ill for a few hours before she died, on the morning of September 17.[146] Cholera was named as the cause and Ann became the first recorded victim of the disease in the colony. At the news of her mother-in-law's sudden death, Francis Mary rushed to Nassau with her one-year-old daughter in hand to bury her.[147] It was the beginning of a coming flood of funerals, as cholera erupted in the Eastern Parade area.

The man who opened the hatches of the *Reform* became an early cholera victim. His sickness was blamed on having inhaled the stale air from the hold of the ship.[148] The disease then spread to the Eastern District. This residential area and voting constituency began about a quarter mile east of Hall Lane. Chipman described it as a jungle bush rimmed by a long line of houses that faced the harbour, which belonged to fisherman and wreckers, their vessels at anchor nearby.[149] On Sunday, September 19, twenty-four-year-old Rachel Armbrister became the district's first cholera victim. As was typical, her illness lasted just a few hours.[150]

On Monday, September 20, the day Captain Evans took the *Reform* out on a wrecking mission, cholera killed Mrs Sara Melissa Brice, 52, and Mrs David Sears. Mrs Brice's son, George Albert, 17, died of the disease a few days later.[151] Mrs Sears' daughter, Emily Susan, 22, a St Andrew's Presbyterian Church Sunday School teacher and a 'gentle and unobtrusive soul', also fell victim.[152]

The first news in print of the cholera outbreak appeared on September 22, when both *The Nassau Guardian* and the *Bahama Herald* carried it as their lead story, along with emergency notices from the Board of Health. 'Since our last issue', began *The Nassau Guardian*, 'cholera has made its appearance in the swamp parts of the Eastern District, and has proved fatal in many instances, the number of deaths being as we understand, 14 out of 33'. The *Bahama Herald* counted even more cases.

> It is with extreme regret that we have to announce the existence of a severe form of cholera in our hitherto healthy Island. The first intimation we received of this fearful visitation was on Saturday last, when two fatal cases transpired. Up to the time we go to press we have ascertained that 36 cases and 17 deaths have occurred, being nearly 50 per cent of those attacked. Hitherto the pestilence has been confined to one locality in the Eastern District,

> known as the 'White Ground' or 'Swamp,' and we trust that there be a strict observance of the sanitary regulations, which are recommended in this publication by authority, and by the blessing of God thereon, the destroyer may be stayed.[153]

Terror spread in New Providence with the news of eighteen persons killed in just five days. *The Nassau Guardian*'s editor parroted the maxim that strong emotions, like fear, increased susceptibility to the disease. This placed the public in a Catch-22. He wrote the following.

> Since unusually healthy as our island generally is, the sudden outbreak of the distemper has created a great deal of alarm. That such should be the immediate effect we cannot be surprised, but we were truly astonished at the widespread panic which everywhere prevailed on Monday. This was judged just as dangerous. Experience has amply proved that there is scarcely anything which more predisposes a person to take the disease than the fear of it. Many, we believe, have died from that cause alone. We cannot, therefore, too strongly condemn the uncontrolled indulgence of this feeling. Besides, for those who lived in healthy localities, there was no good ground of alarm. The epidemic is known rarely to assail persons of regular habits and robust constitutions, breathing a pure atmosphere. An impure one not only generates disease, but will aggravate all kinds of it. Can it, then, be at all surprising that with the heavy showers

> of rain of the past week, which, after a very hot and dry summer, have deluged the very marshy Eastern District, should have produced sickness of some kind among its inhabitants? Certainly not. It was a result to be anticipated.[154]

The misguided moralisation continued.

> Whatever may be the especial character of the disease, we cannot too strongly press upon our readers the extreme danger, – yea the folly, the insanity of yielding to useless fears.
>
> Moreover, there has been a very sensible abatement in it. The weather has fortunately become sunny and fine. We trust it will remain so, and that ere our next impression the epidemic will have disappeared,

The sun came out and the editor ventured that the disease would now disappear, 'through the merciful intervention of Divine Providence'. But damp air and wet ground did not cause cholera and it would not be dispelled by drying soil and sunny skies.

The newspapers demonstrated civic responsibility in sharing guidance on how to manage the disease, drawn from the accepted wisdom of the day. The remedies devised were, in the main, nonsensical and would have been laughable had they not been both unpleasant and harmful. One well-meaning citizen recommended the newspaper the advice given in *Modern Domestic Medicine*, a popular home medical guide.[155] Its prescription for cholera began as follows.

> The first step which we would advise, would be the placing of the patient in a warm bed where he is to be chafed with hot flannels all over the body, while a hot bath is preparing. The flannels might be impregnated with ardent spirits and hot water, as soon as procured, substituted for the dry flannel. Meantime we would administer 3 grains of opium and 10 grains of calomel instantly, followed by moderate potations of warm brandy and water, while the skin is cold, and the circulation concentrated about the internal organs. We would be inclined to repeat 3 grains of calomel and 2 of opium every two or three hours, till reaction took place, and the tide of circulation flowed to the surface. As soon as the bath was ready, we would place the patient in it, having put a good allowance of salt and mustard in the water. If by these means heat be restored on the skin, and the spasms and vomiting be allayed, the great danger is over and the management of the feverish reaction requires but very moderate skill. The injection of 50 or 100 drops of Battley's sedative,[156] or common laudanum, in a small quantity of starch or gruel, into the rectum, might be beneficial.[157]

The list of medicines recommended in the 1827 (third) edition of *Modern Domestic Medicine* amounted to what doctors today call shotgun therapy. It advocated chicken broth, barley water, toast water, toasted oat bread and, of course, generous doses of opium. Irritant concoctions of camphor, pepper, mustard powder and ammonia and spirits of nitre, which the FDA finally banned completely in 1980, were on the list. Magnesium carbonate, a laxative antacid, was also hyped as a therapy that had saved 'many hundred lives in India'. However, it admitted that if, after all this, rubbing the skin with hot wet and dry towels and dosing the patient with mercury and opium while in a hot bath failed, then the case was hopeless. It dismissed the 'complicated machinery of practical medicine, recommended by some, more from speculation than otherwise', as a waste of time and energy.[158]

Days after cholera began sickening and killing White residents in the Town and Eastern Districts of New Providence, cases were being reported Over-the-Hill in Grants and Bain Towns. Immediately, it was clear that this was a serious outbreak. Church bells were tolling at a rate never before heard and obituary notices began appearing in every edition of the thrice-weekly newspapers, where before there had scarcely been one or two a month. Before long, cases were being reported all the way out at the settlements of liberated Africans at Carmichael and Adelaide, some twelve miles distant. Chipman announced that the disease went everywhere that it was invited by filth and 'other localising causes'.[159]

By September 25, when Captain John Robert Hall returned, New Providence was in the grip of the epidemic.[160] *The Nassau Guardian* named the eight White citizens of New Providence killed by the disease in October; John W. Jones, Samuel Griffin, Thomas Pritchard, Miss Esther Butler Claxton, aged 52, and Mr William Mather, a 38-year-old Ordnance Yard foreman, were the first five.[161] They were followed by Glorvina Polhemus, 16, Charlotte Mary Ann Wood, 15, and sister, Mary Jane, 21-years-old. Glorvina was the youngest daughter of Mr John Polhemus. The newspapers informed that they shared a mother, but that

Charlotte's father was the late Honourable George Wood, while Mary Jane, who was married to a 1st West India Regiment lieutenant, was the daughter of John Peabody Patterson, M.D., a Royal Navy surgeon.[162]

On September 20, even before the epidemic reached Over-the-Hill, Lieutenant Governor Nesbitt took his first two decisive steps to meet the epidemic. First, he professionalised what had been a lay-majority Board of Health. 'In consequence of the unhealthy state of the Eastern District', he invited the doctors Kirkwood, Chipman and Duncome, along with Hugh Mackey, staff-surgeon to the garrison, to serve. They consented and were appointed with immediate effect.[163] Had Clutsam not been away, he too would likely have been appointed to the Board. Nesbitt's second decisive step was to call an emergency meeting of the Executive Council. When it met on September 21, it had before it the new Board of Health's recommendations on the immediate actions needed to care for the sick and to stem the spread of the epidemic.

The Board urged finding a house to be used as a cholera hospital, initially referred to as a 'Depot', to which patients in need could be taken. The Depot would have 'proper nurses' and a 'proper person to keep an account of persons applying for aid, and to distribute medicine, food and other appliances ordered by the physicians and to supervise the nurses'.

In a move that the government would come to regret, at this emergency meeting the Council handed the Board of Health the sweeping authority to 'adopt *any* immediate measures necessary without any great delay and *without reference to the Governor-in-Council*'.[164]

At the same meeting, the Council ordered the immediate closure of St Matthew's Northern and Middle Burial Grounds. New grounds would have to be quickly found because bodies for burial were arriving at a frightening pace. The Council directed that the search be concentrated between Baillou Hills and Grants Town, meaning as far from the town of Nassau as practicable. In the meantime, it supported the Board's advice that lime be thrown on top of each corpse in the grave before it was closed. The engineer was ordered to secure a sufficient supply for this purpose. The emergency meeting of the Council also addressed the panic that was being spread by the incessant tolling of church bells. Everyone could hear that a calamity of epic proportions was unfolding and the Council wanted the sounding stopped. It ordered churches to discontinue the practice.[165]

The new Board of Health began to meet almost daily. At its very first meeting, it prepared a public notice of lifestyle measures that the public needed to be aware of to prevent cholera. C. G. Whylly, secretary to the Board, saw to it that the information was published repeatedly in *The Nassau Guardian,* beginning September 25.

> Cleanliness of person as well as of your houses and premises. The cold or tepid bath, as usual when convenient. Every kind of filth or impurity should be removed from the premises and lime freely used in privies, and etc. The keeping of hogs

> should be discontinued for a time least, they being a source of filth.
>
> Avoid overcrowding of apartments, only a limited number of persons should be allowed to occupy one apartment, especially during the hours of sleep. Free ventilation should be practiced when the weather is favourable, by keeping doors and windows open.
>
> Clothing should be warm, particularly in the morning and evening; wear flannel next the skin, and a tight bandage of the same material around the body. Keep the feet warm and dry; observe regular hours, and avoid unnecessary fatigue. Avoid intemperance and excess of every kind. A single drunken fit may be the predisposing cause of a fatal attack.
>
> Food. Diet should consist of solids rather than fluids. Moderation should be observed in eating and drinking, and the interval between meals should not be too protracted. It is not necessary to change your ordinary diet, but be careful what you know agrees with you. The free use of common salt and cayenne pepper is beneficial – the former being highly recommended as a preventative. Fluids: avoid all liquids – cider, ginger beer and lemonade, and ardent spirits.[166]

At one of its early meetings, the Board recommended a ban on the importation of fruits and vegetables that looked 'unsound'. Secretary Whylly, who had signed on to what he must have thought would be a sleepy position, was overwhelmed. The epidemic blew up the position into a programme of too-frequent and increasingly tense meetings, correspondence and notices to be prepared for publication. He resigned and the post went to one Alexander Thompson, who would become the hardest-working secretary of any Board of Health in the history of the colony, although he would have to wait until November 3 to be formally installed.

Of course, none of the recommended treatment-preventative measures recommended by the Board worked. And in any event, who among the poor was in a position to avoid sleeping in an overcrowded house? Who could give up the keeping of hogs? The Board's advice came over as impractical and elitist, and it was clearly failing. Families were losing multiple members within hours. In one home, it was said that a man and his wife were found dead in bed with an infant suckling its mother's breast. Public gatherings were cancelled and friends stopped shaking hands; even persons who appeared to be in mourning were shunned. Individuals began to refuse to go anywhere near a cholera victim, causing the sick to be abandoned.[167] People were left to die isolated and alone, as would happen again in a twenty-first-century epidemic.

John, an old church warden, shared a striking memory of the time. Likely muddied after seventy-plus years of telling and retelling, his story took the form of the parable of the Good Samaritan.

> While the plague was raging, I had occasion to go on a short distance from the town. I took a hack to make the journey as quickly as possible. It was not long before I was breathing the pure air in the open country, and just as I was about to return towards the town I met a clergyman, the father of a

> numerous family. He, like many others, had fled from the fatal contagion; yet still, he was a pious soul, of a very exemplary character and an all-round good Christian to his flock. He preached to them with sincerity and eloquence, but in spite of all, in the hour of danger, he fled – not so much for himself; his family were alarmed by the panic and he felt he must go with them.[168]

The fleeing clergyman was told that in town, 'the doctors are discharging most nobly their glorious mission', but he continued on his way. At noon one day, another cleric, who had remained in the thick of the epidemic, encountered a gaggle of workmen while he was doing house-to-house visits. They had surrounded a man who was lying on the ground, violently sick. The workmen merely gawked, too frightened to help. The clergyman forced his way through with a wheelbarrow, lifted the man in and took him to the nearest medical station.

Persons like the caring cleric that Bethell described in this 1937 account were not altogether rare. *The Nassau Guardian* praised the actions of the 'many excellent private persons' who were providing and distributing supplies. The commissioners of the New Providence Asylum chipped in, making cloth and blankets, corn, sugar, rice and coffee or tea available for collection at the Asylum at no charge. The institution remained adamant, however, that no individual with any infectious disease could be admitted.[169]

The Board of Health admonished those who were distancing themselves from the dead and the dying. In a formal notice, it stated the following.

> As Cholera has not been found to be contagious from personal intercourse, it is hoped that no parties will shrink from doing their duty to their sick friends and neighbours, and to the dead; and not disgrace themselves by contrary conduct.

This position was arrived at after considerable contemplation. Chipman, for one, had agonised over the unknown aspects of cholera and its transmission. He weighed the evidence, comparing it with typhus and scarlet and yellow fevers – all seemingly related diseases, thought to be caused by an unknown poison: 'The poison which ordinarily, when not so rife, not so virulent, shows itself in lesser degrees, in the shape of intermittent, in stronger is remittent, and in its somewhat more potent influence, yellow fever, and in its most powerful, cholera.' The medical men on the Board agreed that the disease was not contagious and that the doctrine of contagion was harmful.

> We all of the profession strenuously opposed the idea of contagion; and, by our example, I trust we carried out the idea that cholera is not contagious. Fearful as has been the havoc which the disease has made, I believe the coolness, and disregard to the doctrine of contagion, has saved many lives; and, on this account, such a belief should not be admitted without the most decisive testimony. II, etc.[170]

The Board's ignorance and contradictions became evident as the epidemic unfolded. Its about-face on the handling (or the avoidance of handling) of cholera corpses did nothing to inspire public confidence.

❦ ❦ ❦

Cholera home remedies promoted by laymen included garlic, tobacco smoking, vinegar sprinkled about the house and bags of camphor hung around the neck.[171] They were much better than those recommended by the experts, which were much worse than useless. The depth of doctors' ignorance is shown by their inclusion of laxatives like castor oil and Gregory's mixture (a preparation of rhubarb, ginger and magnesia), which made no sense whatsoever. They declared that the diarrhoea of cholera was easily cured if treatment was started at the outset. Twenty drops of laudanum (10-per-cent opium powder in alcohol) and camphor, washed down with brandy, was to be the first line of defence. Repeated dosing every two hours until the diarrhoea stopped was recommended.

Any patient dosed with the amount of opium that the cholera prescription directed would soon have come under a hypnotic haze. However, sufferers in this weakened state were not permitted to die peacefully. When diarrhoea continued, doctors blamed the patient for not beginning treatment soon enough and they urged caregivers to force the patient to consume a concoction of camphor, calomel and cayenne pepper mixed with gruel, along with more opium. A brew of chalk, carbonate soda, camphor, ginger and laudanum might also be tried. The onset of painful leg cramps, which indicated severe dehydration, would be treated with quinine (the effective agent and still used by some today) and mustard, but not fluids. Patients too ill to stand were warmed, rubbed and wrapped in cloths soaked in turpentine.

The well-meaning doctors were oblivious to the actual cause of the cramps and collapse in a cholera patient. In reality, the smorgasbord of remedies they pushed through the Board of Health amounted to a form of benevolent homicide (see Appendix 1).

❧ ❧ ❧

The Board of Health's fear that rotting vegetables could produce the inhaled poison that caused cholera led to recommendations on their importation. Lieutenant Governor Nesbitt gave its advice the force of a government order. At the beginning of October, the public was informed that produce arriving in the colony now had to be in perfect condition before it could be taken to market and sold. A certificate attesting to the healthy condition of the produce had to be received before it could be landed, and this certificate had to be signed by a majority of the members of the Board of Health.

Something of this nature would normally be under the sole purview of the port health officer, but for some reason, in this instance his authority was weakened. The order stated that any blemished produce could not be marked down and sold, but had to be taken away (not dumped in the harbour) and destroyed.[172]

The practicality of this new order was immediately tested when, on the evening of Sunday, September 26, Captain Robert Dorritie sailed the brigantine *Pedraza* into Nassau harbour.[173] The 140-ton Philadelphia-made vessel arrived from New York with a shipment of 1,390 cabbages. The following morning, James Black, the port health officer, inspected the vessel, her crew and cargo. He condemned the whole shipment of cabbages, worth some

$97.30, declaring them 'unfit for food, as they are undergoing fermentation, and must therefore be very unwholesome.'[174]

Black ordered Captain Dorritie's shipment to be taken to Salt Cay and buried at the high-water mark. Dorritie, who was part-owner of the cargo and now out-of-pocket, was livid. He marched over to the offices of Drs Kirkwood and Chipman and convinced them to come and see the condemned cabbages for themselves. The doctors did so straight away. That very day they fired off an opposing opinion. What they wrote demonstrated how little they respected Dr Black.

> We the undersigned members of the Board of Health, this day inspected the cabbages alluded to by James Black, Health Officer, in his notification next to the certificate, and considering them in as good and sound a condition as cabbages ever are when imported from America, and with the exception of small portions of the external leaves, are not undergoing any fermentation whatever, or any other process which would render them unfit for food; in fine, they are in a good marketable condition. W. Kirkwood, MD. HN Chipman MD. September 27, 1852.[175]

On September 28, the lieutenant governor chaired the second meeting of the Executive Council following the outbreak of cholera (see Appendix 6). At the table was the George C. Anderson (attorney general), William Vesey Munnings (provost marshal), Felix MacCarthy (police magistrate), John G. Anderson (receiver-general) and Robert A. Thomson. Management of the epidemic was the only item on the agenda.

The sobering first-week statistics showing that 117 cases and 34 deaths had already been recorded were presented.[176] The Board of Health had communicated an emphatic position that no cholera patients should be admitted to the New Providence Asylum or the African Hospital. The establishment of cholera hospitals in Bain and Grants Towns was recommended and the Council allocated £200 to rent and set up suitable houses for this purpose. It also ratified the Board of Health's call for a prohibition on the importation of 'unsound' vegetables and halted the sale of ice. A final item tabled was Reverend L. Swann's offer for the use of his school premises in Bain Town as a depot for the distribution of food and clothing during the epidemic, and it was welcomed.[177]

Within a fortnight the Board had opened cholera hospitals in eastern New Providence and in Bain Town. The eastern hospital operated for just two weeks, closed, reopened and then closed for good before the year ended. It appears that the Board elected to concentrate its efforts at Bain Town and the hospital envisioned for Grants Town was never established.

❦ ❦ ❦

In just two weeks, the colony went from business-as-usual to having the deadliest September on record. In October 1852, the Board of Health began releasing statistics. The first numbers appeared on October 2 and were updated weekly. The first week's statistics appeared along with the lieutenant governor's optimistic assertion that the mortality rate was only 25 per cent and 'less than the general average'.

The Executive Council met that very day to address new problems. Great difficulty was being experienced in finding graves for cholera victims and there was a severe shortage of manpower to dig new ones. The Council turned to prison labour; inmates who had been sentenced to hard labour would be brought out to help dig graves.

The Council met again on October 5 and at this session the lieutenant governor aired his anxiety over the rapidly mounting expenses to the colony's cash-strapped Treasury. Of particular concern were the charges being run up by the government's payment of £2.2s a day to each of the three doctors temporarily hired by the Board of Health. In addition, he was alarmed at the expected cost for all the medicines that were being used on the poor – medicines that ought to have been sourced from the Public Dispensary but were coming from a private pharmacy.

The government had issued only three private pharmacy licences in New Providence: one to a Thomas Brice, another to Dr Kirkwood and the third to the joint owners of the Apothecaries Hall.[178] A fine of £20 for each infraction awaited anyone lacking a licence who dared to retail 'any drug, medicine or any preparation' other than castor oil.

Apothecaries Hall was a standalone private pharmacy on Frederick Street co-owned by Drs Chipman, Duncome and Black. It sold various items, like effervescent magnesia, cod-liver oil, chamomile pills, tooth powder and soap.[179] It also happened to have all the medicines that the doctors needed to treat cholera.

Kirkwood, as director of the Public Dispensary, was being paid £40 a year (reduced by £20 from the original amount at its founding) to oversee the facility. The lieutenant governor had demanded an explanation from Kirkwood on the use of Apothecaries Hall for medicine for the poor and he requested sight of the Dispensary's quarterly accounts. At the October 5 meeting of the Council, Kirkwood's answer was read into the Minutes and subsequently published in *The Nassau Guardian*.[180]

> Sir, I have not furnished any quarterly accounts for medicines furnished for the public use during the last quarter partly because I have been extremely busy and partly because I am in doubt whether any instructions have been given to Mr. Duncome, Black, and Chipman, to supply the public cholera hospitals and the poor generally with medicines from the Apothecaries Hall, which they have been and are now doing, and as it may be presumed, that they not do so gratuitously, but on the contrary, charge the usual shop prices to the public. I am anxious to ascertain if any orders to authorise these proceedings have been given, as, if the law relative to the supply of medicines to public establishments is to be nullified on one side that I may have the benefit of such nullification on my side also, by charging the same as other parties. I have the honor to be, your obedient servant, W.M. Kirkwood, Physician to the Public Dispensary. October 2, 1852.

The Council called on the owners of Apothecaries Hall to clarify how they came to be suppliers of medicines to the poor at public depots and the cholera hospitals. Chipman defended the pharmacy co-owners with the position that the Board of Health had authorised them to get what was needed from their pharmacy.

It turned out that they were in fact acting within the bounds of the government's emergency orders. The lieutenant governor himself had appointed the doctors to the Board and he had assigned to it the responsibility for all public expenditure related to the epidemic. Chipman pointed out that the lieutenant governor had given the Board emergency powers to spend without reference to himself or the Council. Nesbitt was forced to concede that while no specific authority had been given for its doctors to use their private pharmacy, the urgency of the epidemic caused this 'departure from the normal practice'.[181] The Council would move to close this lucrative loophole but not before it had been exploited to the fullest.

At this same October 5 meeting, the lieutenant governor raised the possibility of employing Hector Gavin, the West Indies medical inspector, to help the colony get a grip on the epidemic. Considering the advice that the inspector had put together for the authorities in Trinidad, he thought that he would be well worth his fee of £3.3s a day. The Council deferred to the Board of Health for its advice on the matter.

Just days after the Council meeting, the Board of Health returned an emphatic 'No!' to the question of employing the medical inspector. Chipman and Duncome, whose work the inspector would be coming to oversee, had attended the same medical school as Gavin. As far as they were concerned, a doctor who would be coming to observe and to advise the government but not to personally treat cholera cases was not the kind of help they needed.

The awful tally of deaths from cholera continued to appear in

*The Nassau Guardian*, causing the colony to turn to prayer. With the support of the government, ministers of the various denominations set October 7 as a National Day of Prayer and Humiliation 'before Almighty God, in consequence of the awful pestilence with which it has pleased Him, in his inscrutable wisdom, at present to visit us'.[182] The public was urged to participate, 'by ceasing from their ordinary worldly callings, so that day may prove in every respect, one of solemn humiliation before God, and that He may, in mercy, avert the plague from their habitations'.

Throughout the nineteenth century, the racial segregation of The Bahamas extended to worship in church. Three denominations of the Christian Church were represented in the Over-the-Hill community: Anglican, Methodist and Baptist. St Agnes Anglican Church was a new house of worship at the time of the epidemic. Only consecrated in 1848, the establishment was the handiwork of Reverend William J. Woodcock (1818–1851), an English solicitor who was himself the son of a priest.

Woodcock had previously visited The Bahamas in search of relief from his tuberculosis and had fallen in love with Grants Town. His condition improved and he went back to England, only to return again as a priest. The archdeacon assigned him to the Cure of St Agnes, which comprised the 3,000 persons who lived in Grants and Bain Town. Woodcock directed his intellect to improving education for former Black Bahamians.[183] He used his own money to purchase the property at the corner of Market and Cockburn Streets, where a schoolhouse was built that became the Woodcock Foundation Schools.[184] Black people were welcomed and involved at St Agnes, unlike at Christ Church in the heart of Nassau Town or at St Matthews, at Nassau Town's eastern limit, where they were merely tolerated.[185] Pews at Christ Church were rented to paying parishioners, a fundraising strategy that protected its members from having to sit next to humble citizens.[186]

The Methodist Church had been represented in Over-the-Hill since 1839 in the form of Grant's Town Chapel. In the year of the epidemic, the Chapel gained a new pastor, William English. His flock were not barred from Ebenezer on Shirley Street or the Methodist Church on Harbour Island, but there Black people were expected to enter by a side door and to sit in the rear.

The Baptist Church was the largest and oldest of the Over-the-Hill denominations. All of its members were Black and resided in the Grants and Bain Town suburbs. The accord demonstrated among the denominations over the Day of Prayer was of recent vintage. For years they had been at odds, principally over the Anglicans' control of public cemeteries. The massive increase in corpses and dwindling space would test the durability of the legally mandated truce between the denominations.

Nassau's active public cemeteries comprised the Eastern Cemetery, Bethlehem and the Western Cemetery, or Potters Field. The Eastern Cemetery consisted of three sections; on the waterfront facing Hog Island, at what is today the threshold of the beach soccer stadium, was the Northern Burial Ground. It was designated for Black people and persons of colour only until 1833, when the governor ordered the clergy to no longer use race distinctions in burial grounds. It opened in the 1730s, at the same time as the Centre Burial Ground, located on the south side of East Bay Street. Centre Burial Ground remains but is inactive. The cemetery that grew around St Matthew's Church became the largest section of the Eastern Cemetery and is still in use today.[187]

Bethlehem Burial Ground was located at the northern edge of the Over-the-Hill community, at the top of the New Providence ridge. Soil cover there was thin and its graves had to be dug into solid limestone. Few of its graves could have been more than four feet deep. The growth of Delancey Town at the western edge of Nassau placed the cemetery in the midst of the community. Alexander Bain (1812–1891), who lived on Augusta Street in Delancey Town and who had given his name to Bain Town, became the most prominent permanent occupant of Bethlehem. In the early twentieth century, the site was made a public park with a part of the grounds incorporated into the Willard Patton Preschool, but Bain's monument remains there.

In 1826, the Bishop of Jamaica visited New Providence and consecrated these burial grounds. His act cemented the authority of the Anglican Church over the grounds, whose control included the exercise of demeaning rules, one of the most contentious of which was the requirement that non-Anglican clergy step aside upon the arrival of a funeral cortege and allow an Anglican clergyman to conclude the service.[188] Despite the fact that the public cemeteries had been purchased and maintained from the public purse, no Presbyterian, Baptist or Methodist minister was permitted to conduct a graveside service. The rule led to shameful graveside clashes.

Appeals had been made to successive governors for compromise, but the Reverend Dr John McCammon Trew, archdeacon of Nassau, refused to give an inch. The controversy remained a hot potato until 1850, when under the administration of Governor Gregory, a new Act at last removed the archdeacon's exclusive privilege over graveside burials.[189] Notwithstanding the Act, the Anglican Church retained significant powers over burials. Christ Church Vestry controlled the price for the digging of graves, which it set at 8s.4d each, and it controlled the cost of hiring a hearse. This had been an 'exorbitant charge' of over £1 until January 1851, when it was reduced to 16s.8d 'dressed' and 8s.4d 'plain'.[190] On top of this, Archdeacon Trew dragged his feet in complying with the new Act and this influenced all of the clergy. It caused the Lord Bishop of Jamaica to make a special trip to Nassau to urge his clergy to fall in line. He was conscious of the fact their stubbornness only further drove the ongoing effort to diminish Anglican control over the colony's affairs.[191] These efforts were evident just six months before the epidemic, when a bill to abolish the annual government stipend of £93 that the Anglican Church enjoyed for divine services at St Mary's was read for the second time in the House of Assembly. 'It is high time', said the Honorable Member for Crooked Island, 'for all churches to pay the expenses of carrying on their own worship'.[192] The bill was defeated but the push for reform continued, culminating in the Disestablishment Act of 1869. However, in the third week of the epidemic, when the official death toll stood at ninety-eight, all clergy were swamped by the demand for officiants at funerals.

Archdeacon Trew settled the problem for his denomination by

invoking a rarely used provision for deputising laymen. He authorised vestries to delegate persons to preside over burial services. The composition of the deputies, drawn from parish vestries, revealed just how closely Church and State were intertwined.[193] Christ Church appointed Thomas Williams, W. E. Armbrister, J. A. Brook and John B. Burnside. St Matthew's appointed the Honourable William Munnings, who was a member of the Executive Council, and Nathaniel Webb, superintendent of the New Providence Asylum. St Anne's appointees included the Honourable George Campbell Anderson (1805–1884).[194] This powerful official, who appropriately lived at the top of Parliament Street, was simultaneously the sitting Member of Parliament for the Eastern District, the attorney general, a member of the Executive Council and Speaker of the House of Assembly, a chair he occupied for a record-breaking thirty years. John Minns, a former slave and a baker who lived on Union Street (now called Elizabeth Avenue) in Grants Town, was a remarkable standout as the only Black man to be appointed.[195]

Baptists, Methodists and especially Presbyterians had fought long and hard to win the right to bury their own flock. They now witnessed how a privilege denied to the clergy of their faith was handed to Anglican laymen with a stroke of the archdeacon's pen. Yet, in the midst of the epidemic, annoyance provoked by the archdeacon's action quickly became secondary to the problem of where all the bodies would go.

The earliest cholera victims were buried straightaway. James Ross, the sexton at St Matthews, had his hands full. The dead of every denomination were buried in the cemetery he maintained and he was called out day and night to each interment. Ross attempted to give each corpse a decent burial, an impossibility without help. He pleaded with the vestry for an assistant and, being refused, he paid a William Minus as a helper out of his own pocket. It was the only way to cope. The men obtained and positioned some 200 gravestones to mark the cholera graves – not the typical flat-slab headstones, but short cuboid blocks painted black. With disease all around and working non-stop, it is little wonder that Ross himself fell ill.[196]

Within a fortnight, all of the prepared graves in all of the cemeteries were filled. An all-out effort began to dig new graves and to prepare old ones for reuse. The difficulties increased when the Executive Council, acting on the advice of the Board of Health, issued a series of orders that showed how greatly officials feared cholera spreading from the dead to the living. It ordered the Northern and Middle (or Centre) Burial Grounds closed, while insisting that corpses be in the ground and sprinkled with quicklime within twelve hours of death.[197] A few days later it compounded the problem by prohibiting the reuse of graves as an additional precaution.[198] At the same time that officials were telling people not to shrink from caring for the sick, their pronouncements were sending the message that cholera could jump from the dead to the living.

John B. Burnside, a Christ Church vestryman, reported the difficulty with gravedigging being experienced at the Bethlehem Burial Ground. A prison gang along with four paid stonecutters had been working there from morning till dark, and at the rate they were going they would never be able to dig enough graves.

More men were needed, but people were too afraid to work near a cholera corpse and no additional help could be found.

Softer ground to dig into had to be located, Burnside implored, or bodies would be left unburied. He suggested Hog Island and sought immediate authorisation to dig there from Felix MacCarthy, the police magistrate and chairman of the Prison Committee. MacCarthy dashed to get the lieutenant governor's approval. On the night of October 9, he made his way to Nesbitt's home and handed an urgent message to the guard, with instructions that His Excellency be troubled to read it straightaway. It read as follows.

> Sir, I have now to apologize for troubling you at this late hour of the evening, but I think it my duty, without delay, to make you aware of the following facts, which have come to my knowledge. The gang of prisoners returned this evening from Bethlehem Burial Ground. The overseers report that they have dug three graves today, which have been already filled. When they were leaving the ground, there were two coffins deposited there, for which there were no graves, and the contractor had gone to fetch another. There were no field labourers at work and unless some steps are taken to provide graves, these three bodies are likely to remain unburied until Monday. Under the circumstances, to prevent any accumulation of unburied bodies, I would respectfully suggest to your honor the expediency of taking such of the prisoners as may be willing, out to work tomorrow. In my humble opinion, as a choice of evils, it is better, in this emergency, to work on the Sunday

> than to leave the dead unburied. In connection with the subject may I mention that the place now used for burial for the cholera district, vis., Bethlehem, is very badly suited for the purpose. It is all of solid rock as hard as flint. I am not aware of any better land up on this island but I am informed that there is very good ground at Hog Island, where four or five graves could be dug with as much ease as one in Bethlehem. In conclusion, I have to state that, should I receive your Honor's authority to do so, I will personally see to the employment tomorrow, of the prisoners, and I beg also to tender my services in having graves dug on Hog Island, if it should appear in the morning (which I fear will be the case) that the number of deaths are such that it will be impossible to continue to dig graves in the rocky ground at Bethlehem. I remain Your Honor's most obedient servant, F. MacCarthy.[199]

Nesbitt, awed by the magnitude of the unfolding disaster, immediately authorised MacCarthy to take a prison gang out to work on Sundays and approved graves to be dug in the sandy ground on Hog Island, 'as far from the Town of Nassau as may be', and at Silver Cay.

Two days later, Burnside reported on the progress at Hog Island. The team had completed several burials, having found it easy to dig down to five and a half feet in the sandy soil on the ridge overlooking Cabbage Beach. They had taken every precaution to have 'as little exposure of the coffins as possible'. This meant, no doubt, that coffins were unceremoniously dumped in the holes and hurriedly covered.[200]

On October 13, the Executive Council ratified the governor's go-ahead for burials on Hog Island. It never occurred to the Council to run the action by the Board of Health.[201] When the Board got wind of what had been done, it practically convulsed. Clearly the officials who had approved this madness had no idea of the danger they had created. A gentle sea breeze blowing over the beach and sandy graves could now bring air laden with cholera poison to the mainland. The Board fired off an objection, which the government had published in *The Nassau Guardian* for 'general information'.

> Sir, I am directed by the Board of Health to request that you will be good enough to acquaint His Honor the Lieutenant-Governor that the Board having seen with much surprise and regret, that graves are being dug on Hog Island for the interment of persons dying with cholera, are of the opinion that the pursuance of this practice will be most injurious in many respects, and the Board most strongly recommend its discontinuance, and recommend that a suitable place to the westward of the Town be chosen for a place of interment; for instance, the Sand Bank immediately to the north of Fort Charlotte, or the Bank below the Tea House. A. J. Thomson, Acting Secretary, Board of Health. October 11, 1852.[202]

The Council immediately backtracked and halted Hog Island burials. Initially, the Council rejected the Board of Health's suggestion to use the land north of Fort Charlotte and appointed a committee to urgently find a location for a new burial ground.

The committee, comprising MacCarthy and Mathews, revisited the Board of Health's recommendations and within days it was reported that 'a piece of land is about being purchased at the westward for a burial ground'.[203] With another fifty-three deaths from cholera in just the preceding five days, they had no time to waste.

❦ ❦ ❦

While care of the dead was causing consternation, the Board of Health had its hands full attending to the living. Its emergency measures were proving more expensive than predicted and the Board was forced to inform the lieutenant governor that it was running low on both supplies and funds. The irritated acting commander-in-chief clamped down. On October 11, he coopted the trusty MacCarthy and three members of his Executive Council (G. C. Anderson, Webb and Munnings), along with John S. George and Stephen Dillet, to form a new committee named the Auxiliary Board of Relief.[204] This newborn bureaucracy was tasked to 'guard against the abuse of the public charity'. Henceforth, anyone needing medicine or supplies who was unable to pay would have to present their case for scrutiny.

The Auxiliary Board hired a clerk, a Mr John Ritchie, and on weekdays between the hours of 9:00 a.m. and 3:00 p.m. he sat in the Committee Room of the House of Assembly to receive applications for relief from the public. The mere requirement of a written application, and one that had to be delivered to the House of Assembly, was a significant hurdle. Who would help the illiterate person to write it and who could take time off to deliver it? Without a doubt, this new measure put the brakes on the doling out of public assistance.

❦ ❦ ❦

On October 13, the lieutenant governor again pressed the idea of employing the West Indies medical inspector. Gavin was still in Trinidad, where he had recently investigated an epidemic of diarrhoea that turned out to be dysentery and not cholera. Nesbitt showed the Council Gavin's impressive report on cholera prevention in Trinidad, which he had received earlier in the year. Someone had also sent a copy of the report to *The Nassau Guardian* and its editor highlighted the *San Fernando Gazette*'s commentary on it. 'It ought to be read, and kept as a text book by everyone who desires to aid in improving the condition of his fellow man in the island; by everyone who is called on in any way to discharge official duties to the public, for there is scarcely any department which has not some duties bearing more or less upon sanitary questions.' Dr Gavin's report was very much on target where it stated the following.

> It is enough to remark, that epidemic cholera cannot be kept out by quarantine, and that it has been now sufficiently often confessed by governments of the Colonies in the West Indies, and of the coast of South America, that epidemic yellow fever can be stopped by no quarantine, cordon, or regulations, but only by sanitary improvements directed to the drainage of certain localities, and the affective cleansing and ventilation. Hector Gavin MD.[205]

This insight contrasted with the assertion made elsewhere in Gavin's report that the mortality of almost 30 per cent of children under five years of age among the poor in Port of Spain was due to 'the ignorance, carelessness, and fondness of pleasure of parents in that class'.

When the Executive Council met on October 26, it faced new challenges in addition to the Board of Health's plea for more money. Reverend Whitehouse had complained about the macabre sight of dead bodies bouncing about in the open carts that were being used to haul them to the burial grounds. The Council sent £200 to the Board and ordered the civil engineer to find a covered cart for the transportation of corpses.

Letters from seven Out Islands had come in pleading for medicines and supplies. The Council requisitioned pieces of flannel and cases of medicines from the New Providence Asylum for distribution. It hired three 'small sailboats' that took them to Abaco, Andros, Eleuthera, Grand Bahama, the Berry Islands, Bimini and Grand Cay. Its final bit of business at this meeting was to make a payment of almost £25 to the civil engineer for the work of clearing bush in the Eastern District and in Grants and Bain Towns.

The supplemental funds given to the Board of Health were quickly spent. At the Council's very next meeting, on November 2, it appealed for and was given additional funding. It had spent £504 (approximately $73,000 today) since the onset of the epidemic, including £184 in October alone. And as if the present epidemic of cholera was not worry enough, word reached the Council that yellow fever had broken out in Charleston.

The volume of shipping traffic between Charleston and New Providence made an outbreak of disease there a serious concern. The Council ordered that all ships arriving from Charleston were to fly a yellow flag. This was a major a departure from the normal practice, where a yellow flag was required to be flown only when disease was known to be on board. The Council also reiterated the colony's standing rule that one was not allowed to disembark a vessel arriving from outside the colony until they had been cleared by the health officer. In making this pronouncement, Charleston and its yellow fever outbreak were singled out for mention. Before the year was out, that city would have cause to reciprocate the cold shoulder and hold up traffic arriving from New Providence.

An account by a Delancey Town shopkeeper, written during the height of the epidemic, has survived. Henry Stevenson, the son-in-law of Charles Farquharson, penned it on October 14, 1852. Farquharson's journal is considered a national treasure.[206] Stevenson's family, the O'Briens, were well-known residents of Hospital Lane and it is likely that his Delancey Town shop was very close by.

> Dear Brother (in-law), I write you these few lines hopeing [*sic*] that they may find, and all yours, Enjoying good heath [*sic*], you may have heard before [?] that the Cholera has made its appearance here [?] and has been commiting [*sic*]

great ravages: it commenced at the Eastward ½ and carried off a great many and then shifted down to Bains town, and then in grants town and then up towards us. Miss Braynan [*sic*] opposite us died last Saturday it has been all around us both at home in, the Bottom and at the Shop – thank God none belonging to us has had it yet, and we pray that if consistent with the will of the Almighty we may be spared. all [*sic*] your family is well as yet; as well as ourselves – the deaths has been from 6 a day to sixteen which [*sic*] as far as I have heard, your sister charlotte [*sic*] has returned from Inagua – she is very ill – the doctor has seen her and does not think that she will Survive but, a few weeks – we heard from Andros Island that this week your Sister was not very well, I think she might have been up had she not heard of the Cholera – will you tell Mrs. Dickson that her Brother – old daddy Tom is dead – he died of this disease – poor old man I hear that Death was very welcome to him, and that he died very happy – you see we now in truth in the midst of death all around us, Still we trust in the mercy of our God – weather [*sic*] we live or die – With regard to the house, you seem to wish that I should repair it, and, take the rent until the Expences are paid up – I had reathe [*sic*] make some arrangement for the purchas [*sic*] of it – if we could lower to terms about It. that [*sic*] is if the thing could be done, is in this uncertain StateIdont [*sic*] Know what is [?] take placeIdont [*sic*] Know if the thing is pratcable [*sic*], I will see after it in the mean time and let you Know, I have not been able to get anything from Mrs. Thorne, as she has not received any money from home from some cause or

> other, yet – nor has I teer [?] Smith about the money that he owes you. Since writing the above cholera has risen yet more & more – it has not got in town, we are all trembling for ourselves not knowing when we may be Called yet we hope in God. I hope there may be soon another chove [?] to Watlings when if I am spared I shall write you again [?] time I remain yours. Henry Stevenson.[207]

If Stevenson saw comfort or benefit in the strategies of prevention or the treatments offered by the Board of Health, he made no mention of them. He felt that he was completely at God's mercy. The government would not directly admit its powerlessness, but within days Lieutenant Governor Nesbitt and his Council sanctioned another day of fasting and prayer.

The early-November numbers on the epidemic gave hope that the prayers were being answered. The pace of new cases in New Providence appeared to be slackening. Still, a dark mood hung over the island, as if a beloved head of state had died. So many families had been decimated that everyone appeared to be in mourning. The wealthy had stopped their afternoon buggy drives. The markets that normally bustled with buyers were as dead as the day after a hurricane. The produce grown in the African settlements of Sandilands, Carmichael and Adelaide 'by the industrious Nangoes' was nowhere to be found.[208]

Nesbitt had held the governor's seat on several occasions in the past, but this time around he probably wished that he was the one away on vacation. Governor Gregory's six months' leave were up in October. What was taking him so long?

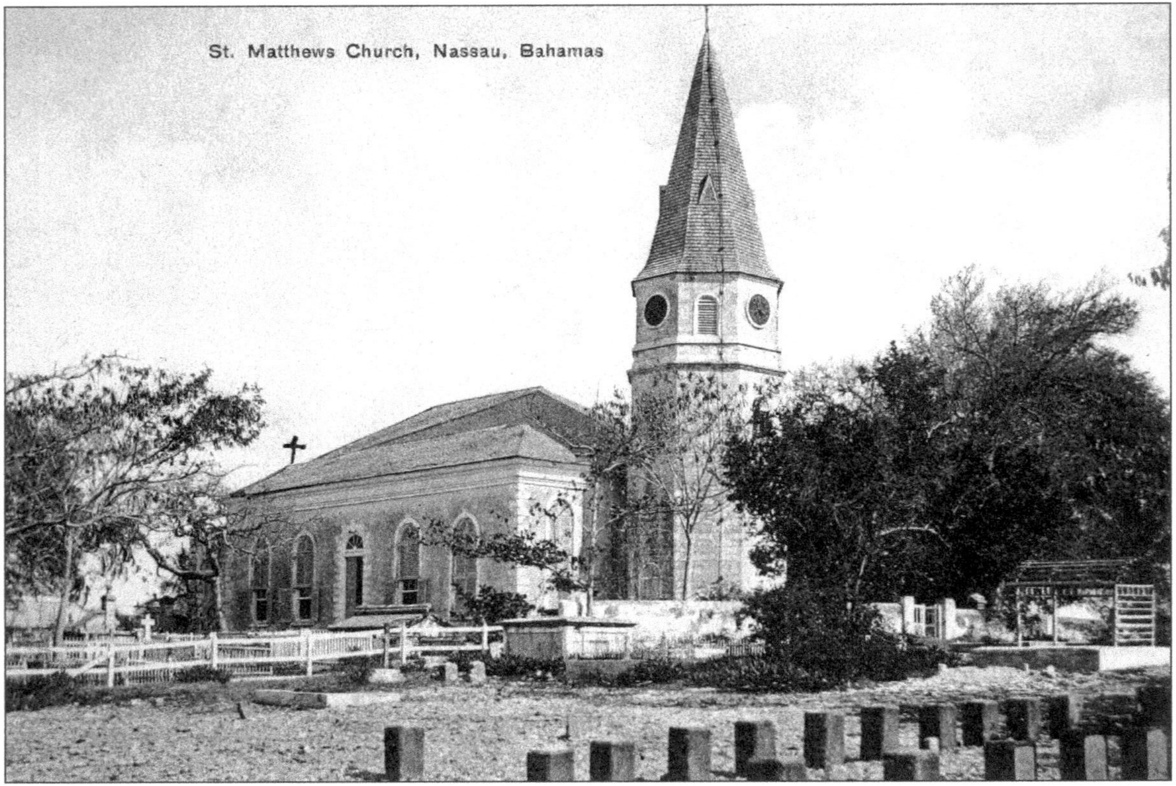


1. 4. St Matthew's Church Graveyard, 1914. Cholera stones in the foreground. Courtesy of Captain Paul Aranha

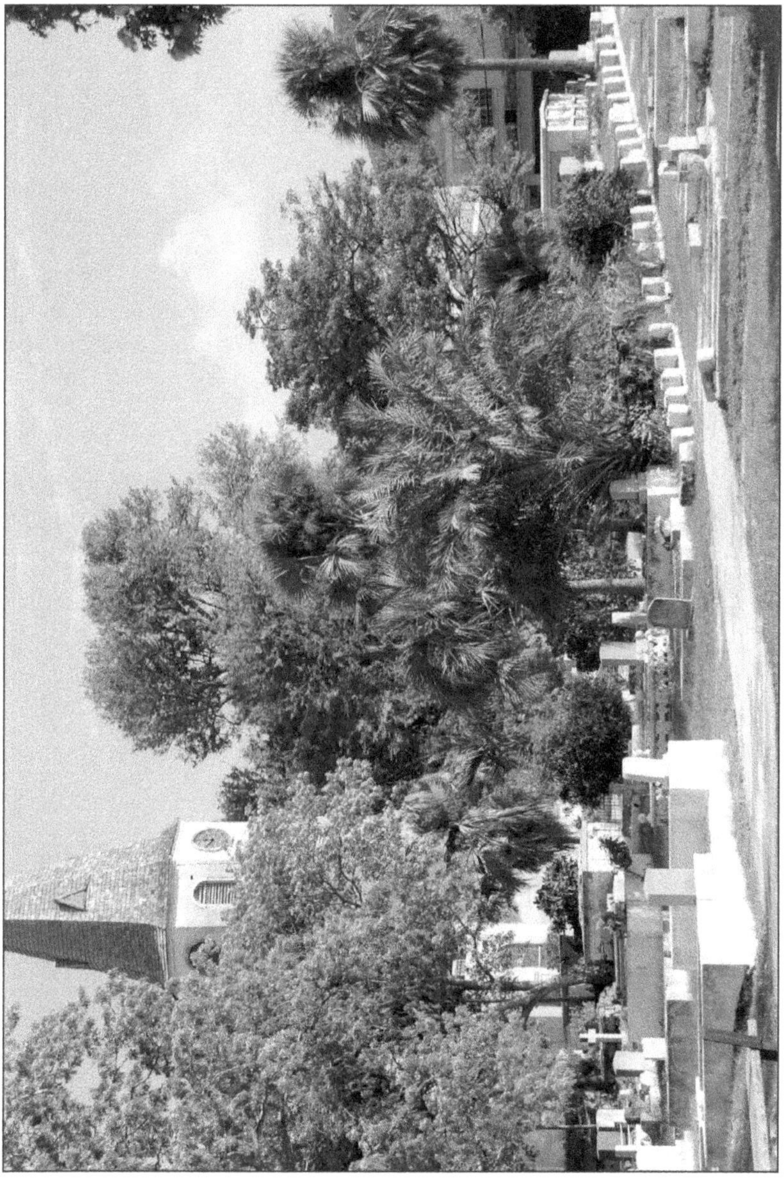

*5. St Matthew's Church Graveyard, 2014. Cholera stones lining the walkway. Author's photograph*

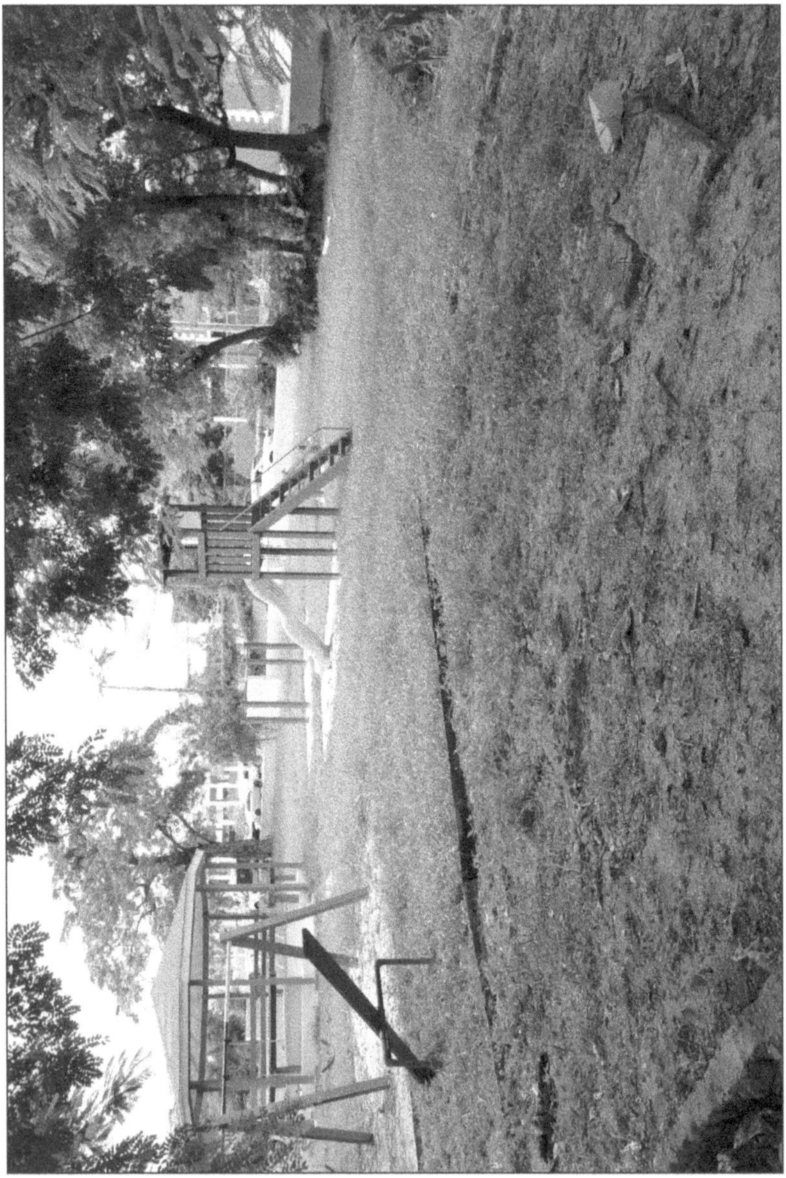

6. *Bethlehem Graveyard/Public Park, Meeting Street, New Providence. Author's photograph, 2023*

# 4

## Gregory, Gavin and Farre

On the evening of November 7, 1852, a loud swoosh followed by a window-rattling bang over the town of Nassau caught the attention of residents who were just sitting down to Sunday dinner. Anyone outside who looked up would have seen a display that lit up the evening sky. The lieutenant governor knew straightaway that it was a signal, fired from the Royal Mail Steamship *Esk,* an indication that Governor Gregory was aboard. Officials scrambled to complete last-minute preparations to receive him and the Ordinance Wharf answered with a rocket of its own. By 6 p.m., when the *Esk* dropped anchor, Legislative and Executive Councilmen had changed into appropriate attire and were hastening to the dock. Ordinary residents thronged to the waterfront as well. The flurry of activity surrounding the governor's return and the government's demonstration of his importance was welcome entertainment in the normally quiet town. Dinner would have to wait.[209]

Gregory's journey back to the colony from England had begun

on *La Plata,* a Royal Mail paddle steamer. He was travelling with his wife, his two daughters Henrietta Charlotte and Louisa, his four-year-old son Philip, two female domestics and a manservant.[210] The party had a three-day layover in St Thomas, the hub that had linked Europe with the Americas since the 1840s, when the Royal Mail Steam Packet Company negotiated permission from the Danish government, which 'owned' the island. Its fine harbour – the finest, it was said, in all the Caribbean – was a dangerous place for visitors. The island was rife with yellow fever.

West Indies Medical Inspector Hector Gavin met the governor's party in St Thomas. He arrived, manservant in tow, just in time to board for the trip to Nassau. Their conveyance, the 232-ton RMS *Esk*, was smaller than *La Plata* but she sported the new-style steam-powered screw propeller. The *Esk* had been brought into service in 1849, and at her normal cruise speed of eight or nine knots the run to Nassau took five days.[211] At 112 feet in length, she carried twenty-nine passengers, if they were packed like sardines. Even at half of maximum capacity, there would not have been much space. *The Nassau Guardian*'s editor mused on her comfort: 'Esk – the tidy little Esk, whose accommodations are modelled on the scale of the black hole of Calcutta, sent once to Demerara as a floating prison for those who had committed the enormity of paying their passage to the company.'[212]

The voyage to Nassau soured within hours of departure, when Gavin's servant fell ill with generalised aches and a fever. The following morning, Midshipman Van Runim developed the same symptoms. Over the next three or four days, five more sailors, including Burnett, Young and William Vincent, came down with yellow fever. Vincent, 18, was the ship's second officer and, notwithstanding his youth, the Falmouth teenager was practically revered by the crew. Only a few months earlier, he had been a midshipman, but not on the *Esk*. His entry to the ranks began aboard the ill-fated RMS *Amazon*.[213]

On January 2, 1852, the *Amazon* departed Southampton on her maiden voyage, bound for St Thomas. She was several miles out when she caught fire and, in what survivors described as an horrific scene, 104 persons drowned or burned to death. Survivors described Vincent's actions as heroic and were adamant that the death toll would have been much higher had it not been for him. Vincent's employer, the Royal Mail Steam Packet Company, informed Queen Victoria and the young man was summoned to the palace to receive Her Majesty's personal congratulations. In addition to his audience with the sovereign, the Company presented Vincent with a gold watch and a promotion. Until now, his rapid elevation to full command had been virtually assured; however, at this moment, the life of the teenager who lay groaning on his swaying sickbed was in grave danger. Charlotte Gregory and a family servant also fell ill with yellow fever. Gregory thanked the Almighty that Dr Gavin was aboard, and he watched in awe and with gratitude as the physician ministered to his family and the crew. The *Esk* became a floating hospital, and when she dropped anchor in Nassau, Vincent was in critical condition.

The *Esk* broke all of the rules on entry to the colony. The captain disregarded the regulation that ships with known or suspected yellow fever on board must fly a yellow flag and, contrary to the regulations, when the port health officer boarded, he was not alone. Kirkwood joined him, closely followed by Chipman and Duncome. While the medical men conferred over what to do with the governor and his party, another thirty bigwigs climbed aboard, hanging around until the doctors came to a decision. They announced that quarantine was unnecessary and cleared Gregory and company to disembark.[214] Undoubtedly, the doctors would have denied having felt under any kind of pressure when they short-circuited the established protocol.

Gregory feigned surprise and dismay that he was allowed off. In his first report back to the Colonial Office he alleged that he had been fully prepared to submit to quarantine and that he had even urged the doctors not to give him special treatment.[215] Nonetheless, the courtesy afforded by the experts suited him just fine. His daughter was seriously ill when she was hurried from the *Esk* to Government House. Kirkwood took over her care from Gavin and soon after being put to bed she brought up the dreaded foul-smelling black vomit. The sick seamen were held on board until the following morning. Vincent, Van Runim, Young and Burnett were taken to Mrs Hudson's inn, opposite Government House. While there, under Dr Chipman's care, each of the men in turn manifested intestinal bleeding: black vomit.[216]

Gavin also lodged at Mrs Hudson's with no special precautions and no fear of contracting yellow fever. The very next morning, he was at the governor's door. He handed the commander-in-chief a letter that began as follows.

> Your Excellency, I have the honour to state for the information of your Excellency that I received at Trinidad on

> the 27th ultimo a Despatch from the Lieutenant Governor of this Colony dated 12 October and that having submitted this Despatch to His Excellency Lord Harris and after consultation with His Excellency I considered it my duty to proceed forthwith by the Return Packet to this Colony. I have now to report my arrival last evening to your Excellency. In conformity with my instructions I have to produce to Your Excellency the accompanying letter and my instructions. I have also to submit to your Excellency the accompanying correspondence in relation to my prolonged stay in the West Indies with a view to Your Excellency taking such steps thereupon as to Your Excellency may appear expedient. I would also place before your Excellency a copy of my Despatch to H. M. Undersecretary of State for the Colonies on my proceeding to the Bahamas.[217]

Gavin invited the governor to appoint him to the Board of Health 'so that I might the more readily carry out the instructions which I have received from Her Majesty's Government.'

Two days after their arrival, Officer Vincent died at the inn. He was buried in Potters Field with military honours.[218] Vincent and his fellow crewmen, along with Charlotte Gregory and the other *Esk* passengers, were the first yellow fever fatalities the colony had seen in seven years.

The governor acted on Gavin's suggestion with speed and on November 10 appointed him to the Board of Health. Gregory was aware that the Board had opposed Gavin's engagement and that the doctor had come without a formal invitation. None of this mattered to the governor after just having shared such a harrowing journey. It became even easier to sweep aside resistance when Gavin presented his credentials, which showed he was there on the authority of Her Majesty's Government. To his colleagues on the Executive Council, Gregory cited the high quality of the report that Gavin had produced for Trinidad as the deciding factor. The governor-in-council employed him immediately at the rate of £3.3s per day.

❦ ❦ ❦

The governor's first despatch to Sir John Pakington reflected shock and awe at the scale of death that had preceded his return to the colony. More than 600 souls had been taken in the first month and a half of the epidemic, and some weeks saw an average of thirteen deaths daily. In October, a record twenty-eight deaths occurred in a single day, and on the day he returned, Dunmore Town alone had twenty deaths. The respect and gratitude he held for Gavin was clear in his communique.

> I have the honour to report that I arrived here from England at 6 o'clock on the evening of Sunday the 7th instant and resumed the administration of the government of the Bahama Islands on the following morning. I need not describe my feelings as the governor of the colony when I learned of the distressing condition to which it had been reduced during the last six weeks by the ravages of Asiatic cholera. The whole population of the island of New

> Providence is little more than 8,000, yet in the short space of six weeks this fatal disease has carried off between 600 and 700 persons. The largest number of deaths in any one day has been 28, the next largest 26, the highest average per day 13. The average of the last days, seven. By far the largest number of persons attacked have been black or colored, but the white portion of the population has not escaped. There are four medical men in Nassau, three of them are physicians and one is a surgeon and a general practitioner. All of these gentlemen have been placed upon the Board of Health and their personal exertions have been laudably, indeed, almost incredibly great. Such have been the exertions of the clergy and the ministers of religion of all denominations.[219]

The governor shared that he had been oblivious to the cholera epidemic in the colony until he was returning from vacation.

> I first heard of our misfortunes on 31 October, when I arrived at Saint Thomas, and it was a source of great satisfaction to me to find there Dr. Gavin, who quitted Trinidad the moment he heard of the cholera having appeared in the Bahamas, and was then on his way to Nassau. He accompanied me in the small screw steamer *Esk*, and most providential it was, as we had not been out to sea above 24 hours, for the yellow fever broke out amongst the crew. That the Royal Steam Packet Company have not deemed it their duty to place a medical man aboard the *Esk*, you can at once judge the sorry state to which we would have

> been reduced had Dr. Gavin not been with us. The medicine, which the captain had on board, was of the simplest kind and wholly unsuited to our circumstances. My own medicine chest contained the most extensive articles and under the blessing of God, with the able professional exertions of Dr. Gavin, we reached Nassau without any death occurring on board. Not so however, when we landed. For the count of the next 36 hours, one of the officers of the *Esk* died, and I am in hourly expectation of hearing that two other cases have terminated fatally. We have also two very serious cases in Government House; my eldest daughter and one of my female servants. And if the language of this despatch should appear to you to partake of a character somewhat inconsistent with the usual tone of official communication, I must beg of you to excuse it and attribute it to the natural anxiety of a parent attendant a large family.
>
> Since I commenced this despatch, the two cases under my own eye have undergone a very favourable change and I am greatly relieved.[220]

In the same despatch Gregory feigned innocence in breaking the regulations. The strengthened Quarantine Act that he had a hand in enacting just eight months earlier called for quarantine when any passenger or crew was even thought to suffer from any contagious disease. It was enacted primarily to keep the colony free from cholera, yellow fever and smallpox. How convenient it was that all of the medical men in the colony suddenly agreed that yellow fever was not contagious and that quarantine was unnecessary. Practically everywhere else, including in England, the accepted wisdom was that yellow fever was contagious and that quarantine was required.[221]

Once comfortably reinstalled in Government House, he shared with the Colonial Office that he immediately became aware that there were many persons in the community who were displeased, if not fuming, that the *Esk* had not been placed in quarantine. The move flung the port open and authorities could no longer in good conscience enforce quarantine on any ship with yellow fever aboard. This was in evidence the following day, when a ship arrived in New Providence with her captain seriously ill. The governor wrote the following.

> The day after we arrived here, another vessel arrived from St. Thomas and the master of her is now lying dangerously ill with the same disease as that which the *Esk* has unfortunately brought to the colony. My own opinion from the first breaking out of yellow fever on board the *Esk* was that we should be placed in quarantine on our arrival here, but such was not the opinion of the Health Officer, or of Dr Gavin, or of Dr Kirkwood. I earnestly entreated these gentlemen to decide the question without the slightest reference to the accidental circumstance of the Governor and his family being on board, and I took care to address them in the most public manner on the question, and indicated that I was quite prepared to undergo the most rigorous quarantine, if the health officer, acting under the quarantine laws of the colony, should think it fit to order the *Esk* to the Quarantine

> Ground. To my surprise, the three medical men, after personally visiting the six cases of yellow fever then on board, unanimously declared it to be their opinion that the disease was not contagious or infectious and consequently that there was no need whatsoever for subjecting us to quarantine. I accordingly forthwith landed, and brought the sick members of my household to Government House, where every possible attention has been paid to them by Dr. Kirkwood. A few days will solve the problem whether the yellow fever, thus brought to our shores, will or will not spread through the community. If the medical men prove to be good prophets, I shall be only too happy, but, on the other hand, if my own fears, in which a large number of persons participate, should prove to be too well founded, I shall at least have the satisfaction of reflecting that I am in no degree whatever responsible for the consequences of the *Esk* having been admitted at once to free pratique. I am well aware, nor can I be surprised, that a vast amount of dissatisfaction exists in the community at the moment, in consequence of this importation of yellow fever and I doubt that you will not concur and I that I owed it to myself as the Governor of the colony to take every legitimate opportunity of removing from my own shoulders the responsibility attached to the act of admitting us to pratique.[222]

The prevailing cholera epidemic quickly subsumed worry about the introduction of yellow fever. The current emergency had brought commerce to a halt. It had caused a widespread and paralysing fear in both White and Black residents but, according to Gregory, only the labouring class, meaning Black people, panicked. His prejudice that they were easily frightened was widely held.[223]

> Since the breaking out of cholera six week ago the colony has suffered lamentably in all its interests; commercial and social. For the first fortnight there seems to have been a perfect paralysis amongst all classes of people. No supplies of meat, fish, fruit or vegetables were brought to the market, and the labouring portion of the population seem to have been struck down by a species of panic. Things however, are now improving. The disease itself appears to be decidedly on the decline. The general gloom is wearing off, and I entertain a sanguine hope that by the mail of next month I shall have the satisfaction of reporting the cessation of this formidable disease, at least in the island of New Providence. I much fear however, that the numerous islands, of which the Bahamas Government is composed, will each in turn, be visited by cholera. It has already appeared in Harbour Island, adjoining Eleuthera, and at the Bimini Islands, opposite the coast of Florida. Inagua has hitherto been free from it but I can scarcely hope that this exemption will long continue.[224]

Gregory appealled for the remuneration of Dr Gavin and revealed the circumstances of the medical inspector's engagement.

> Before I close this despatch, I would venture to exert my hope that under the distressing circumstances by which the Bahama Islands are now surrounded, the Lord

> Commissioners of Her Majesty will consent to make provision for the whole of the salary and traveling expenses of Dr. Gavin while he remains here. I am aware that under a recent arrangement, a moiety of his salary shall be paid by the colony which he visits, but in the present case, Dr. Gavin was not invited to come, for Lieutenant Governor Nesbitt discovered that the Board of Health saw no receptivity for such an invitation being lent and he consequently abstained from doing more than apprising Dr. Gavin of the fact of cholera having made its appearance here. The result was that, with the concurrence of Lord Harris, he proceeded to Nassau and most glad I am that he did so. I placed him immediately on the Board of Health and have only seen him once since we landed, for with his well-known zeal, he has devoted every hour to the public service. Our revenue is at all times very slender, but under the existing circumstances of the colony, with a very heavy expenditure going on for the relief of the sick poor, I am very conscious of our inability to pay Dr. Gavin for his services as he is entitled to be paid. I would therefore earnestly recommend that he should be permitted to draw the whole of his salary from the date of his departure from Trinidad to his return thither. I have the honour to be sir, your most obedient, humble servant. John Gregory.

Gavin matched the governor's early report home with one of his own. In his first of several to the Earl of Desart, the under-secretary of state for the colonies, the inspector indicated how quickly he had gone to work and taken charge.

> I attended a meeting of the Board of Health at 12 noon on the 8th, stated my views as to the means of prevention necessary and then visited part of the infected Districts. On the 9th I submitted various resolutions to the Board which were forthwith adopted and forwarded to His Excellency for his approval and that of the Council – and again visited parts of the infected Districts. On the 10th I presented the Schedules, Instructions, Notifications etc. for the approval of the Board of Health, which were ordered to be printed. I have endeavoured to acquire some more precise knowledge as to the extent of the epidemic and efficiency of the measures of prevention taken. I am unable to afford any information as to the extent of the disease of so accurate a character as to be depended upon, but, I believe I am nearly correct in stating that about five hundred or more deaths have occurred in New Providence. I regret to add that, notwithstanding the zeal and earnest desires of the local medical men a great number of persons must have perished without medical aid whatever.[225]

No statistics were yet available for the Out Islands but the disease was known to be in Harbour Island, Andros, Exuma, Bimini and Grand Bahama. By November 20, the Board of Health's official tally was 1,485 cases and 501 deaths, and most of those were from Grants and Bain Towns. Yet while the loss of Ida Blanche, the thirty-week-old daughter of the English commander of the West India garrison, made the newspapers in November, not a single one of the Black citizens who were dying in droves Over-the-Hill were named in print.[226] *The Nassau Guardian* did not, however, fail to report on October 30 that Justice Mathews had sentenced Peter McDonald, William Gilcot, Joseph Sawyer and Peter Coakley to imprisonment for up to six months for larceny.[227]

Inspector Gavin assured the Colonial Office that he had been well received, and boasted, 'the local medical men are not only willing, but glad of the opportunity to co-operate with me'. He shared the top items on his agenda: the introduction of a systematic programme of house-to-house visitation, and the appointment of nurses and an inspector of nuisances. This was to be a policeman who would check lots and yards for the presence of weeds, stagnant water, rubbish, visible sewage and outside toilets that were not six feet deep. Gavin also wanted to fix how deaths were recorded and communicated.

Having witnessed the death harvest in Grants Town, Gavin was disturbed by the fact that so many persons there had no access to a doctor. He placed addressing this deficiency high on his agenda. He would have community-based medicine depots and dispensaries for the poor established.

Gavin attacked the 'allegation' that the disease had been brought to the colony by the *Reform*, claiming that cholera had been in the colony, 'though not in its severe form', for the past two years and he closed with a postscript that cholera had broken out in New Grenada.[228]

Coming out of the Board of Health's first meeting with Gavin present was a list of five resolutions that it presented to the Executive Council. The Board sought:

1. to be empowered to extend the system of dispensaries and depots for the gratuitous supply of medicines to persons afflicted with cholera and diarrhoea;

2. that the system of house-to-house visitation, by lay visitors, should be applied to the infected districts under the supervision of inspectors;

3. that inspectors of nuisances should be appointed with the powers of police constables, under clause 27 of the Police Act. In England, the Board of Health had this authority;[229]

4. that the registrars of deaths should be instructed to make returns of the deaths in their several districts to the Board of Health daily under the fourth clause of the Registration Act;

5. the the Board should be authorized to appoint, where necessary, nurses to attend poor persons in infected districts.

The 'resolutions' arrived in time for the first meeting of the Executive Council since the governor's return. In attendance was Colonial Secretary Nesbitt, G. C. Anderson and his brother John Grant Anderson (1793–1858), the colony's receiver-general and treasurer, along with William Webb, Felix MacCarthy and William Munnings.[230]

The governor would have given the Board of Health *carte blanche*, now that his esteemed Hector Gavin was on board, but the Council helped him to see sense. It pointed out to Governor Gregory that medicines and the dispensaries had already been expanded for the poor. The councilmen decided to move with caution and to ask the Board for more information on its intentions. How many medicine depots were operating now, and where were they located? What additional ones did the Board think might be needed, and where? On the matter of increasing the number of lay visitors and inspectors, the Council wanted to know the number presently employed by the Board, and at what pay? How many more did it think were needed, and at what cost?

On the question of appointing inspectors of nuisances, the Council envisioned unspecified complications from endowing citizens with the power to issue orders, when they answered not to the leadership of the police force, but to the health authority. In England, local boards of health had certain police powers but the governor-in-council would not countenance this in the colony.[231] It gave the Board the green light to employ more nurses, but the policing of nuisances was kept under the purview of the inspector of police. Constables would be the ones to report on any 'unhealthy accumulations of refuse' found in and around New Providence residences.[232]

The Gavin-led Board of Health's desire to implement a 'correct system' of statistics with the hope of obtaining better information was a laudable aim. However, its request for the tabulators to produce daily tallies, particularly of the complexity Gavin desired, was impractical. The effect of the order, at least from a public standpoint, was the complete opposite of better and timelier information.

The Board of Health had been diligently publishing weekly totals of cholera cases and deaths from September 21 to November 26. It covered the first sixty-seven days of the epidemic and included those cases seen at the Bain Town Cholera Hospital. The three-day moving average number of cases in New Providence showed the fury of the epidemic. The death rate peaked on October 24, when the count stood at 1,000 cases and 350 deaths. At the point when Gavin joined the body and statistics stopped, it had counted 1,436 cases and 510 deaths. The numbers extrapolate out to the year's end to 525 deaths and 1,800 total cases in New Providence – matching the number later reported by the lay visitors (see Appendix 15).

At the end of November, when the new rule for daily counts was implemented, the publication of weekly statistics abruptly stopped. In fact, the Board released no further cholera data whatsoever to the public.

At its November 10 meeting, the Executive Council had just one distraction from its cholera business and it illustrated some of the pressures faced by the port health officer. The master of the brigantine *Hope* had lodged a complaint about Dr Black. The captain was furious at how long his vessel had been held in limbo, to then be denied entry by the health officer. He thought that the officer had signed off on his paperwork, allowing free pratique, but when he read what he had received, he found that 'the document was of such an unusual character as to completely preclude any possibility of entry'. The Council resolved to ask Black for a report.

On November 12, the governor's first despatch to the Colonial Office and Gavin's initial report were mailed together to England via the *Esk* to St Thomas. A few days later, Gavin's fantasy of being in cordial cooperation with his local colleagues collapsed. On November 16, Kirkwood, Chipman and Duncome, along with the Honourable Thomas Mathews and John J. Burnside, resigned *en masse* from the Board of Health. This left only the chief justice and the port health officer on the Board with Gavin.[233] The retiring physicians cited the tremendous demand for their medical services in the community occasioned by the epidemic as the reason for their resignation. Laymen, they stated, could just as well conduct their administrative functions. The governor publicly thanked them for their service and acknowledged the high-minded explanation they provided as the reason for their exit.

> Gentlemen, I am directed by the Governor to state that he has been induced to accept your resignation of your seats at the Board of Health; solely by a consideration that your professional services to the community at large at this trying season, have been, and continue to be, seriously interfered with by constant and unnecessary attention to matters of detail, which can as well be looked after by unprofessional persons.[234]

Unseen by the public were Gavin's manoeuvrings that had precipitated the crisis. In a letter to the governor, he had lambasted the Board of Health and called for an overhaul of its make-up and operation.[235] It had made sound recommendations in the weeks prior to his arrival, he acknowledged, but its recommendations had been bungled or had failed to be completed. He emphasised that the doctors were in the 'onerous and improper' position of carrying out their own administrative decisions. His most impactful criticism was directed at the Board's financial operation, with Gavin pointing out that the doctors on the Board dispensed their own medicine and other supplies to the poor, billed the Board for what was provided and then approved their own payment. He implored the governor to invite them to resign and to place them on a separate and subordinate body. This secondary health board as conceived by Gavin would offer advice to the established Board of Health but would have neither a say in what recommendations were accepted, nor in how they would be carried out.

Gavin claimed to have discussed this with his colleagues and said that they were in complete agreement. He then unveiled a new plan that called for New Providence to be divided up into medical districts, each to be served by a single district medical officer. Each doctor would be paid £2.2s per diem for providing medical care to the poor in their district. He claimed that this too had been readily agreed by his colleagues.

The proposed shake-up was too much for the governor to decide without additional input, and he reached out to Kirkwood, Chipman and Duncome to directly hear their views. They let him know that they were willing to resign from the Board and to give the district medical officer concept a try.[236] The governor then invited Gavin to pitch his project directly to his Council at its next meeting, slated for November 16.

The medical inspector attended the Council meeting as invited and there outlined his proposal. He also restated his request for police powers for the Board of Health. This was denied but the Council did agree to reconstitute the Board along the lines that the inspector had proposed.

Gavin had effectively engineered a coup. This new reality was pressed home in the second part of the 'Thank you for your service' letter from the government to the deposed doctors. Couched in flowery language, the colonial secretary delivered a stinging demotion as he let them know that as far as public health matters were concerned, they were now subordinate to the Gavin-led Board of Health.

> His Excellency, however, desires to record the high sense he entertains of the valuable services you have rendered to the public as Members of the Board of Health since the commencement of the present deplorable epidemic, and the Governor feels perfectly assured that the same untiring zeal for the public good, which is now the theme of universal praise and gratitude in the community, will induce you to give to the newly-constituted Board, the benefit of your recommendations as to any measures which you may deem to be called for, with a view to the preservation of the public health and the abatement of the existing epidemic. [237]

MacCarthy and William Doyle were appointed as replacements on the Board with terms that ran until May 13, 1853, and a few days later the body published the layout of its new health districts. Kirkwood was assigned to the Eastern District, which ran east of Nassau Town as far as Fox Hill and Dunmore Town. Black was assigned to Delancey Town, at the western edge of Nassau, south of Augusta Street to Meadows Street in Bain Town. Duncome had charge of Bain Town south of Meadows Street and Chipman had Grants Town, including Congo Town and the residential area at the back of Fort Fincastle. No physician was assigned to Fox Hill, nor to the villages of Carmichael, Gambier and Adelaide, because they were remote and had relatively few cases. They would be visited as the 'occasion may require'. The town of Nassau, a district bounded east by East Street and west by West Street, and southward from Bay Street to East and West Hill Streets (see Figure 2), was also excluded from coverage by a Board of Health-paid physician because it too had relatively few cases and its residents were not considered poor. The Board also informed the public that its district medical officers were empowered to employ nurses for those in the community that needed them, but the need had to be urgent and the patient had to be '*poor and destitute*'.[238]

Central to Gavin's programme for fighting the cholera epidemic was a system of house-to-house visits. He had enormous confidence in his system; just as doctors today preach that early detection of cancer and other diseases saves lives, so Gavin preached that early detection and treatment of cholera was lifesaving. The Board immediately hired eight laypersons from the community for the job and gave them a crash course on cholera. Gavin instructed them on the stages of the disease, from the onset of diarrhoea to the appearance of symptoms that required a doctor's attention. Their remit reflected the inspector's zeal. Visits were mandated for each house in their area at least twice a day, and preferably thrice, to seek out cholera cases. Patients found with diarrhoea were to be classified into one of three stages of the disease according to the criteria he provided. Visitors were to provide households with information on prevention and treatment of cholera and to distribute medication. Each lay visitor was paid 30s a week, the approximate wages of a skilled tradesman in England, but still far less than was paid to their counterparts in London. On November 13, they began their work in New Providence. For the first ten days they were under Gavin's direct supervision. Chipman assumed oversight through December, while Gavin visited Eleuthera and Harbour Island.

The work of the visitors was difficult, dangerous and undoubtedly traumatic. They had been tasked to count, question and counsel residents who were suffering from a deadly and poorly understood disease. While most people were distancing themselves from the sick, visitors were repeatedly entering the poorest and most unsanitary dwellings. At one point there were only four of them. We cannot say whether the fall-off was all a result of a government cutback or whether some retired from fear, illness or exhaustion.

One must wonder what instructions Gavin gave them for self-preservation. Perhaps they were told to keep doors open, not to breathe too deeply and not to tarry. Today we would counsel hand-washing and forbid the acceptance of offers of food and drink. Such hospitality had to be refused to avoid contracting cholera on an already stressful job.

As November drew to a close, the number of cholera cases in New Providence fell off steeply. Only thirteen deaths from the disease were reported in the final week, compared to thirty-five in the first week[239] and forty-seven in the second.[240] In addition to two deaths from cholera in Carmichael Village,[241] two of those lost in the third week came from a single prominent White family. Amelia Catherine Maura, wife of the Spanish consul, died on November 17 and two days later her daughter-in-law succumbed. His Excellency John Maura Sr was away in Cuba when Amelia died, having left Nassau on August 27. His son John Jr had been deputised as acting consul in his stead. Don Domingo Rodriguez was dispatched on the *Pacific* to Cuba as bearer of the sad news and Ambassador Maura hurried back, landing in Nassau on Saturday, November 20.[242] On November 22, the press named another White victim: Edmund Burnett, a seaman from the steam packet *Esk*.

On November 24, the Board of Health warned the public that the police were now inspecting premises for nuisances. It urged people to avoid getting wet and preached that nothing was more important for the prevention of cholera than an abundant supply of fresh, clean air. The Board made the ridiculous suggestion that the residents of Grants and Bain Towns should leave the low, damp and filthy areas where they lived and move to higher, drier and healthier places.[243] Another notice informed the public that it had closed the temporary cholera hospitals in the Eastern and Western Districts and lime-washed the houses that had been used. The still-needed Bain Town Cholera Hospital was being moved 'to a more central location'.[244]

❧ ❧ ❧

The Bain Town Cholera Hospital opened in the last week of September and remained in operation for fifty-eight days. In addition to providing care to cholera victims, it served as a base of operation for community outreach and house-to-house visitors. The Hospital eventually admitted 137 patients, equally divided between the sexes. Eighty-two of the patients died – a mortality rate of 60 per cent. As with most diseases, the weak, the sickly and the aged were the most likely to succumb.[245]

Details of the care that was rendered at the Hospital exist thanks to the record of Henry William Richard Farre (1799–1882), an Englishman who grew up in a prominent medical family. His father, Dr John Richard Farre, was an ophthalmologist and co-founder of the Royal London Ophthalmic Hospital.[246] His brother, Arthur, was a professor of obstetrics at King's College and Physician Extraordinary to Queen Victoria.[247] His youngest brother, Frederick, was an ophthalmologist like his father and both brothers were active Fellows of the Royal College of Physicians of London.[248]

Henry had himself attended medical school, but he had shunned practice and turned to a footloose lifestyle. In 1837, he went to British North America (now Canada) for two years. In

Montreal, he joined the armed forces as one of the Loyalists who, he said, 'with God's help, saved those fine provinces to Great Britain and its noble Queen at the risk of their lives'. Farre was fifty-one years of age and recently widowed when, in August 1850, he had came to New Providence. He had lodged at a boarding house on Montague Street, possibly chosen because of its sea-bathing facility.

I believe that Farre came to The Bahamas to improve his health, seeking the improvement that a warmer climate, sunshine and sea-bathing could bring. He vociferously promoted the practice while he was here, in a campaign that makes me strongly suspect that he suffered from scrofula.

Tuberculous lymphadenitis, called scrofula in Henry's day, manifests as a lumpy swelling or an abscess on one side of the neck. Doctors drained pus, applied antiseptic bandages and crossed their fingers that it would go away. In 1731, John Lettsom, who promoted bathing in the sea as the most effective treatment for scrofula, founded the Royal Sea Bathing Infirmary in England specifically to treat this disease. He got the idea from the dubious claim that fisherman seldom developed scrofula. Scientific publications buttressed the claim and, despite the frigid bite of England's beaches, sea-bathing became a fad. Resorts sprang up all over the isles and sea-bathing machines became a thing.[249] The Infirmary itself expanded in the 1850s and, by pumping seawater up from the beach, created indoor sea baths.[250]

In New Providence, the affluent followed England's lead and built private sea baths. Farre detailed the inconveniences he endured in procuring the amenity for himself. The sea bath at his boarding house, he complained, was full of sand, and all of the other good ones about were private facilities. He obtained permission from the head of the local militia to use the officers' sea bath facility (perhaps after he shared his record of prior loyal military service). Even that facility drew complaint. It was 'subject to the tides and only thoroughly available at high water'. What was needed, railed Henry, was a floating bath that was usable at all hours and available to the poor.[251] He offered to assist with the procuring of plans for the construction of a public sea bath and he threatened the authorities with a less-than-polite campaign for its completion, should they fail to heed his request.[252]

It was Farre, in July 1852, who reported the swarms of ants in Bain Town. On August 27, 1852, the lieutenant governor appointed him a justice of the peace.[253] The office would have provided him with the opportunity to derive a small income, but within weeks of being sworn in, the cholera epidemic arrived. It proved to be a call to service and Henry stepped up. Frederick described his brother's role as the resident medical superintendent of the Cholera Hospital at Bain's Town, an office that was 'arduous and somewhat dangerous'. His report on the epidemic began with a restatement of the known facts.

> Cholera is stated to have appeared suddenly about the middle of September at Nassau, in New Providence, whence it soon spread to Bain Town, situated in a low valley behind it. The first death occurred on the 16th of that month, and up to October 12th, seventy-nine deaths were reported from this course; but the real number was supposed to exceed 100. The

> disease, though checked in its original locality, spread rapidly over the island, and, by 10 November, the deaths had considerably exceeded 500 at least of which had occurred since October 10th, giving an average of 125 a week, or 18 a day. The mortality then began to diminish, for, on December 2nd, whole number of deaths was estimated at 700, which leaves something less than 100 for the three proceeding weeks. The cases were at this time few and generally mild, those still occasionally fatal; and, even a month later, seven or eight deaths were occurring weekly. The whole population of the island being about nine thousand, that was at east 8 per cent.
>
> The first person attacked was a native white woman; but, during the early prevalence of the disease, it was almost entirely confined to the colored inhabitants, the white people, with the exception of the doctors and the ministers of religion, having fled from the infected localities. But, after a few weeks, the whites were overtaken, and began to suffer also. The history of this pestilence is not unlike that of the first attack of cholera in England, in 1832. A temporary hospital was first opened in the eastern suburbs of Nassau; but the inhabitants having fled, the pestilence soon removed to another district, and the doctors followed in its wake.[254]

Farre continued with more details on the colony's response to the cholera epidemic.

> Another hospital soon afterwards opened in Bain's Town, where thirty-two cases were reported on 30th of September.

> This hospital was kept open fifty-eight days, and received 137 patients, of whom eighty-two died, or sixty percent.
>
> The eastern hospital was closed when the cholera removed to Bain's Town, but was reopened on the 14th of October, the disease having reappeared in its original locality. I have no record of the cases admitted.

Farre noted that some treatments used elsewhere were not employed in The Bahamas.

> No mention is made of the internal use of opium, except by enema, nor of its external use, though the latter is particularly serviceable in the ordinary cholera of the West Indies, and is perfectly free from the ill effects which frequently occur when it is largely administered internally. Venesection is not mentioned, except in one case – a case of collapse. Emetics and purgatives are also passed over in silence, as well as salines and saline injections. Warm baths are rarely used in the West Indies, even as a luxury, and are not mentioned in the hospital arrangements.

A mortality of 40–60 per cent from cholera was typical in Europe, America and the West Indies but the Board of Health blamed the 60-per-cent level at the Bain Town hospital on the public. In a cry that would be echoed by health authorities in subsequent centuries, people were charged with fatally delaying seeking help. 'Too many people were being brought to the hospital beyond all help and in a state of complete collapse.'[255]

Cholera victims who avoided the Bain Town hospital were doing themselves a favour. Its treatments were unpleasant at best. The exact regimen varied from patient to patient but almost everyone was given brandy and opium. Those too weak to drink the concoction were liable to have it administered by enema. Others were dosed with calomel and port wine. External treatments were added or used alone when medications were in short supply. Cramping muscles were rubbed. Bellies were wrapped in turpentine-soaked bandages or painted with irritants strong enough to blister the skin. Farre wrote that patients begged for water and it was 'freely given', but not with the rationale of treating dehydration. It was given 'to relieve the internal heat'.

The scene at the Bain Town hospital is frightful to imagine. Groaning patients in the throes of death, weakened by severe dehydration and experiencing agonising leg cramps, occupied its beds. The suffocating vapour of turpentine permeated the air. Mind-dulling doses of opium were being administered and patients were forced to sit or to lie prone so that cupping glasses could be applied to the spine. Sufferers were given water likely sourced from a contaminated well nearby. It seems fortunate that even 40 per cent escaped with their lives. For the minority who made it to convalescence, a cloying and bitter concoction of chalk and quinine was served.[256]

Farre espoused the mantra proffered by apologists for slavery that dark-skinned people needed White people for their own benefit and protection. He wrote: 'The Negro race are extremely prejudiced and obstinate and were with great difficulty induced to take any medicine. Of the cases brought to the hospital, many had entirely neglected all means of recovery, and eighteen or twenty were dying when brought in.'

Farre was blind to those entirely sound reasons why the Black population would have been reluctant to seek a doctor's care, even without knowing the details of what they would have faced at the hospital. They were still being exploited as an underclass – former slaves who had no say in their government or even in their own personal treatment.[257] And many knew that the treatments were ineffective.

Farre was a little more insightful about the mortality in the Bain Town hospital. He noted that a mortality rate of only 41.5 per cent was reported at St Bartholomew's in London. He wondered whether the higher rate in The Bahamas was because cholera was more virulent in the colony, or because residents were simply less able to survive the disease. Perhaps, he mused, Bahamas residents had a 'lower vitality' from chronic illness and malnutrition. He was also on to something in his suspicion that the location of the hospital contributed to its high death rate.

> I think, at least probable that the mortality was swollen by the nature of the place where the hospital is situated. Bain's Town occupies a low valley behind Nassau, in the vicinity of swampy ground, only three feet above the springs. In moist weather, at sunrise, a heavy mist hangs over the entire hollow, and fever is very prevalent. Nowhere was the disease so fatal as in this valley.

He was right, but for the wrong reason. The whole water table was contaminated. Residents were drinking water laced with cholera *Vibrios*.

Farre's interaction with the establishment was minimal. His name does not appear in the Executive Council Minutes or in Board of Health notices. No other reports mentioned him in relation to cholera. Farre's own reference to the medical inspector was brief, distant and impersonal: 'Dr. Gavin visited Nassau on a tour of inspection during the prevalence of the epidemic.' This was all that he had to say about the West Indies inspector.

❦ ❦ ❦

At the beginning of December, Gregory penned his second report to the Colonial Office in London since the outbreak of cholera. He began as follows.

> I have the greatest satisfaction in reporting that although there are still some few cases of cholera in Nassau or its suburbs, we are fully warranted in believing that this fatal epidemic, as far as the island of New Providence is concerned, has come to a close, and that when the new year opens upon us, we shall be altogether free from it. I arrived here four weeks since and at that time the deaths had diminished from 70 to 35 a week, and now, thank God, I am enabled to state that they are not above 16 or 17 a week.[258]

Gregory praised Gavin's work and indicated that he had allowed him to take control of the Board of Health. He took comfort in the thought that the inspector shared his priority of cost control. As new challenges surfaced and additional requests came in from the Board of Health, the governor would be forced to face the truth that Gavin had not come down from heaven. But for now, Gavin was the governor's golden boy. He wrote the following.

> Dr. Gavin, the Medical Inspector for the West India Colonies has been indefatigable in his exertions, and as Governor of the Islands I cannot adequately describe the obligations we are under to him. He has re-organized the Board of Health and instituted that most useful and salutary system of 'house to house' visitors. He has vigorously taken in hand our whole medical and sanitary expenditure, which owing to the panic which accompanied the epidemic on its first breaking out in September last, has [placed] on my table such appeals from Harbour Island, Gregory Town, Tarpum Bay, Rock Sound, Exuma, Abaco, Berry Islands, Bimini Islands, Grand Bahama, Carrion Crow Harbour, Spanish Wells, Ragged Island and Andros, and that, which is so painful in the matter is the reflection, that it is totally out of my power to meet all their wants.[259]

The governor shared the fear of a food shortage caused by the epidemic.

> The panic throughout these islands has been so great, that the labouring classes have staid [*sic*] in their houses, and allowed their provision grounds to remain uncultivated, the

> result of which will hereafter be a very general dearth of the necessities of life. In the mean time I have taken no steps in this matter without the fullest discussion in Council, and have laid down such stringent rules for the guidance of those to whom corn and four have been leant for distribution, as will (for the future at least) ensure the appropriation of them exclusively to the most indigent and infirm of the unfortunate inhabitants.[260]

Running out of food may have been a worry for the near future, but an immediate concern was a breakdown of law and order in parts of the colony. The governor ended his despatch with the promise to give a full report on the spot of trouble that he was having with the residents of Governor's Harbour in Eleuthera.

> Nor is famine, or the prospect of famine, the only trouble that has grown out of this lamentable epidemic. In several of the islands, such as been the terror of the people, that utterly regardless of the laws or of the admonition of the local Magistrates, they have taken upon themselves to set up a rude species of maritime and land quarantine, and their attempts to enforce it against ships and persons coming from places within these islands or elsewhere wherein cholera exists, they have proceeded to acts of such lawless violence as to have compelled me at last under the advise of the Council to send down a military force to restore order and the dominion of civil laws amongst this misguided population.[261]

Gregory's brief mention of his having to forcefully restore law belied just how tense the situation had become. In a postscript to his despatch, the governor breathed a sigh of relief that all of his family had recovered from the yellow fever contracted in St Thomas. He gave kudos to his medical advisors for their seemingly correct stance on the question of quarantine and put in a final plug for the inspector. 'Dr Gavin and the other physicians were right. My fears were groundless.'[262]

# 5

# Sticks and Stones

In the final month of 1852, New Providence continued to have new cholera cases, but it was no longer a deluge. On December 7, Chipman reported to the *Association Medical Journal* that deaths were down to 'about six or seven per week'. Some 800 had been counted up to November 19, most of whom were poor Black people. Chipman lamented the manpower shortage, which was exacerbated by the loss of the doctor who normally cared for the West India Regiment; he had fallen ill and fled to England, leaving Kirkwood with responsibility for the garrison. Still, Chipman saw a light at the end of the tunnel and he gave thanks to the Almighty. 'How we got through the work', he wrote, 'God only knows, but we were wonderfully preserved during a most arduous duty, which literally occupied us night and day.'[263]

Chipman's trials were not done. Just after Christmas, on Monday, December 27, he lost Sarah Anne, his wife of twenty years and the mother of seven of his children.[264] She died at age thirty-nine, after 'a short but severe illness', the nature of which was not identified and could have been cholera. In his bereavement, Chipman stepped back from his oversight of the lay visitors. He handed the duty back to Gavin and, after a week or so, Gavin rotated their supervision to Doyle and Black.[265]

Gavin himself began to face increasing headwinds and his grip on the Board of Health began to loosen. Even with the governor behind him and occupying a seat on a Board that held emergency powers, he still needed the cooperation of the local physicians. The inspector's disposition for burning bridges resurfaced, appearing first when he chose to issue orders to his colleagues rather than reach out with personal appeals. When they failed to comply with his requests, he shared his frustration with the governor.[266] Gregory himself had to walk a tightrope in the small circle of his administration and he knew better than to insult the doctors with a command that they kowtow to Gavin. In fact, the government began to look for ways to scale back its mounting emergency cholera expenditure at the very moment that the inspector sought to strengthen his public health programme. It would start, thought the Council, by cutting the number of doctors employed by the Board of Health in half.

The four district medical officers were invited to quote for their services to the Board of Health, giving both a daily and a per-patient rate. 'The governor-in-council', sniffed Secretary Nesbitt, would decide 'which of the two modes of remuneration would be likely to be most advantageous to the public interests'.[267]

Chipman, Black, Kirkwood and Duncome balked and closed ranks. They formed the colony's first ever medical association, calling it the Bahama Medical Board, and appointed Frederick

Duncome as secretary. Duncome wrote to the colonial secretary on the association's behalf and indicated that tendering for their services was beneath their profession. They would work without pay, he wrote at the end of November, before they submitted to the indignity of tendering for a job.

The governor's records and the colonial secretary's memory stretched back decades, and history was on the government's side. The secretary served up an embarrassing reminder to the Bahama Board when he recalled that two of its members had previously participated in tendering to provide medical services to the government; one had tendered to care for the troops at the Fort Charlotte Garrison and another had bid to provide care to a travelling detachment of them. The colonial secretary's smooth rebuke stated that no offence was intended, but rather that 'His Excellency felt that he was treading on safe ground', considering that the practice of tendering for medical services was well established in the military in the home country and had been exercised previously in the colony. He also questioned the authority of the newly-formed body to communicate or negotiate on behalf of the doctors, considering that it had not been introduced to, or recognised by, the government previously.

Rather than engage further with the group, the governor simply cancelled the doctors' £2.2s per-diem. If they stuck to their word, for the remainder of the health emergency, the doctors would now be seeing the poor for free.

The disease jumped to the Out Islands and began a fresh harvest of lives. Governor Gregory found himself besieged by cries for help from every corner of the colony. In a despatch to Sir John Pakington, he wrote the following.

> I have now on my table such appeals from Harbour Island, Gregory Town, and Rock Sound, Exuma and Abaco, Berry Islands, Bimini Islands, Spanish Wells and Ragged Island and Andros. And that which is so painful in the matter is the reflection that it is totally out of my power to meet all their wants.[268]

Twenty-five deaths from cholera had been counted in Abaco. Cases were being reported in Andros, Bimini, Steventon and Moss Town in Exuma, Ragged Island, Rum Cay and in St Salvador (now Cat Island). The Board of Health sent a shipment of supplies from the Dispensary to Abaco and Eleuthera. Ragged Island received 'an experienced nurse with medicines and hospital stores'.[269]

If anywhere needed a nurse, it was Ragged Island. This small, salt-producing island, located some 200 miles south-east of New Providence, was home to about 350 residents. Cholera broke out there on November 9 and killed twenty-five people in ten days.

Ragged Islanders benefitted from the attention of four visiting caregivers: Mr and Mrs Joseph Scott, Mr Wilson and an unnamed letter-writer. One of them noted the poverty of the residents. 'Very few have a piece of flannel the size of my hand to rub with, or for any purpose', she wrote. She mused that if poverty in Nassau was anything like that in Ragged Island, it too would have a fearful mortality from the disease. Her description of life in the midst of the epidemic is the best seen from any of the Out Islands.

> I wish to write to you relative to a disease, which has been, I may say, raging since the 9th on which day the first case occurred. It commenced with, and seems to be more fatal to children; several adults, however, died. We imagine it to be cholera, yet there are many circumstances attending it that lead us to doubt whether it really is cholera. Eight adults have died of it and I buried an eighth child today, after which I visited three others lying in a hopeless state. With them it commences and terminates with vomiting and evacuating that white rice watery substance, unaccompanied with any pain, and a great thirst continues till death terminates the sufferings.[270]

Her description of her experience tending the sick brims with clinical detail.

> The adults are seized [simultaneously] with one or both of these symptoms; the use of the medicines sent from the Dispensary succeed in checking one or both of these ricey discharges; then the difficulty is to keep them generally warm, which we have in many cases managed with all the disadvantages; but notwithstanding the establishment of general heat, they die without any pain, and when *we* think they are convalescing. Many will not keep on their covering,

> such as it is, and those who may be in profuse perspiration in the body, have their extremities icy cold. Some few have been taken with cramp in legs and pain in stomach, the latter has given way to the mixture sent from Nassau.[271]

Before her letter could even be printed, word arrived that Joseph Scott, one of the caregivers, had died of cholera, 'in the very midst of his philanthropic labours'.

One hundred miles to the north-east, on Rum Cay, cholera cut down another White man; William Horne Gould, the twenty-five-year-old revenue officer stationed there, died of the disease.[272] In December on Ragged Island, the Reverend W. H. Strombom lost both his wife, Maria, and his daughter, Fanny Jane, to cholera.[273]

Help and hope came for other islands with the arrival of two physicians aboard the *Pedraza* from Philadelphia: Samuel Joseph Clutsam and a Dr Hall. Clutsam, the native son of a Bristol mariner, was returning home. Before Emancipation, he had been the Member of Parliament for Eleuthera.[274] Nowadays, he practised in Nassau and he provided some services, like smallpox vaccinations, to the poor without charge. But, of late, he was often away.[275] Dr Hall was a newcomer. Governor Gregory reported that he encountered both men by 'mere accident' on November 24 and that he hired them on the spot for two guineas a day each (the same £2.2s received by the Nassau doctors).[276] Clutsam was sent to Eleuthera while Hall boarded the *Globe* for Green Turtle Cay. In the small Abaco community, Hall proved to be a hit.[277] His treatment of cholera cases and his 'urbanity' were so appreciated that residents tried to get him to stay. As his six-week-long engagement approached an end, they drew up a petition urging him to remain. Magistrate Inglis, along with Messrs Hayman and Saunders, spearheaded a fundraiser to sweeten the pot.[278]

In Harbour Island, residents implemented quarantine without official sanction when they heard that cholera had erupted in Nassau. Residents of Governor's Harbour, on the island of Eleuthera, followed suit. Their homespun blockade led to the first military mobilisation of the local West India Regiment seen in many a year.

Cholera hit Harbour Island in its 'halcyon days', that forty-year stretch from the 1840s to the 1880s when Dunmore Town, the island's only settlement, was the second-most important town in The Bahamas.[279] The 1851 Census counted 1,840 persons living in the racially segregated settlement.

The small island off the north coast of Eleuthera had attracted persons to its perfect beaches of powder-fine white-and-pink sand since the 1700s. It began its climb to becoming an economic powerhouse in 1837, when the island was made a port of entry. After 1842, when commonage land in North Eleuthera was granted to hundreds of families, its economy took off. Landowners in Eleuthera turned to fruit-farming and pineapple became their number-one crop.[280] Harbour Island mariners developed boat-building on the island; its shipwrights built bigger vessels than anywhere else in the colony could manage and in 1855 they shipped 36,500-dozen pineapples to the United States.

The count peaked in 1872, just shy of 120,000-dozen.[281] Many Harbour Island mariners also held second jobs as farmers on Eleuthera.

On October 15, 1852, the Executive Council discussed a petition from Harbour Island community leaders who were worried about the epidemic making the jump from New Providence to their Dunmore Town. They were dissatisfied that the government had not enforced or even recommended quarantine on their island.[282] The petitioners implored the governor to expand the quarantine laws to expressly include cholera and they wanted permission to form their own local Board of Health. The Council was surprised to learn through the request that the petitioners had already implemented quarantine on their own. It discussed whether or not to approve the island's unsanctioned actions and, when it came to a vote, the body was divided. Munnings and G. C. Anderson voted 'Ay' and the others 'Nay'. Approval was denied for the Harbour Island quarantine and its leaders were told that, even if it had been approved, the measure could only legally be applied to vessels arriving from outside the colony. Blocking inter-island travel, including from cholera-ridden Nassau, was illegal. Permission was given to form a local Board of Health on Harbour Island, with the wrinkle that the governor himself was to be chairman and its membership was to include at least one justice of the peace. The cost of the about-to-be-formed local Board of Health was of paramount concern and the Council imposed financial controls. The Board would be required to provide an estimate of proposed expenses and it would only be permitted limited emergency costs without the governor's approval. 'Proper accounts and vouchers certified by the local Board' had to be submitted for all expenditure.[283]

Harbour Island's petition and the Executive Council's debate over the island's efforts to prevent an outbreak there proved pointless because the disease appeared there the very next day. The disease erupted simultaneously with its appearance in Bimini, on October 16. Bimini took an early lead, with fifteen reported cases and ten deaths up to October 23, while 'only' five people died of cholera in Dunmore Town in the first week of the epidemic there. Fear of catching the disease quickly bloomed into full-blown panic and those who could fled to Nassau and to Florida, many of them in dangerously overcrowded boats.[284]

Two youthful physicians lived and worked on Harbour Island: Dr Benjamin F. Wendel (1826–1852), 26, and Dr Jeremiah Eneas (1830–1903), who was just 22-years of age. Wendel was a native of Kentucky and a graduate of the University of Louisville. He had spent a year as an assistant physician on the staff of Bellevue Hospital in New York, where he had nearly died after contracting 'ship fever'.[285] In 1850, he moved to Harbour Island, possibly to consolidate his recovery, and he was apparently preparing to return to Kentucky when cholera broke out. He delayed his departure 'to take care of his friends'.[286]

Eneas was a Harbour Island native who in 1850 chose medical school over joining his family's profitable shipping business. He matriculated at the University of Pennsylvania with a fellow Bahamian, George Kemp.[287] Upon completion of his course, he returned to his famously healthy hometown.

Throughout November, Wendel and Eneas were kept busy as

Harbour Island was pummelled by the epidemic. *The Nassau Guardian* of 20 November shared some grim statistics.

> The Schooner *Clyde*, which arrived from Harbour Island today reports the cholera continues in Dunmore Town with unabated violence. Since our last accounts, 35 more persons have fallen victim to the scourge, making a total of 91 deaths up to 11 o'clock yesterday.[288]

The doctors worked around the clock to the point of exhaustion and both of them fell ill during the epidemic. Wendel suffered repeated attacks of diarrhoea but forced himself to return to work the moment he had regained a little strength. Friends feared for his health and pleaded with him to cut back. They watched him go out at all hours of the night, in wind and rainstorms, to visit the sick. 'He had no peace, no rest at home during this cholera, for the people came in dozens for medicine and advice. One day, he looked so thoroughly exhausted and he said, "I have passed such a dreadful time, and if I cannot get sleep I must die!"'[289]

By the end of the first week of December, the official count of cholera deaths on Harbour Island stood at 152. Among the victims was Mrs Walton, the Schoolmaster's wife.[290] Dunmore Town was the only locale in the colony other than New Providence where the concentration of cases led to the creation of a cholera hospital. Caregivers there soon ran short of the useless irritants and life-sapping narcotics that were the normal prescription items. Perhaps more patients there received the basic support and nursing care that they so badly needed. We cannot know this, but we do know that the toll was said to have climbed to 600. Just as the pace of new cases was slackening, yellow fever broke out. Dr Wendel was one of its first victims. Exhausted and weakened by repeated attacks of diarrhoea, he fell ill on December 14 and died just four days later. The terse notice in the Nassau press of his demise also informed the public that Chief Justice Lees had lost his young daughter, Eliza.[291] The cause of her death was not stated and it is entirely possible, if not likely, that she too succumbed to cholera.

Thomas William Johnson was a boy of sixteen years of age when cholera struck his home town. An apocryphal story has him working as a wily doctor during the epidemic; the yarn says that at the end of a workday, he would burn his clothes on a rock and then swim across the harbour to his waterfront home. On the shore, his wife would meet him with a towel and fresh clothes. The system was said to have kept him cholera-free.[292] In fact, young Thomas had not yet gone to medical school, but the epidemic certainly proved a motivator. In 1854, he entered the University of Pennsylvania Medical School. Three years later, with the submission of his final essay, titled 'Acute Rheumatism', he earned his diploma.[293] He returned to Harbour Island and married there at the Wesleyan Chapel in 1860.[294] Johnson served in his home town until his death in October 1895 at the age of sixty. Today, a monument stands in his memory on the corner of Temperance Square in Dunmore Town.[295]

## MISSION TO ELEUTHERA

The island of Eleuthera is located approximately fifty miles north-east of New Providence. It is seventy miles long and not more than two miles wide at any point. The Census of 1851 counted 4,610 persons, and while it was more populous than Harbour Island, residents were spread out over settlements that stretched from Spanish Wells, The Bluff and Lower Bogue in the north, past Governor's Harbour in the middle, to Tarpum Bay and Rock Sound in the south. Clutsam was the sole physician on the island. Normally resident in New Providence, the minute the governor had engaged his services he and his wife, Catherine, had departed for Rock Sound. More than thirty-five deaths from cholera had already been counted between that settlement and the nearby Tarpum Bay when he had set out. Residents were crying for help.

Somehow the settlement of Governor's Harbour, located just twenty-five miles north of Tarpum Bay, was free of cholera, but its residents were rightfully terrified over the approach of the disease. In an effort to remain cholera-free, they copied Harbour Island and implemented their own quarantine without asking for permission from Nassau. On Thursday, November 25, two days before Clutsam reached Rock Sound, the homespun blockade thrown up led to a clash with the central government, triggered by the arrival of Stipendiary Magistrate Carleton, who had travelled to Eleuthera to begin his regular tour of judicial duty.

Carleton and his party sailed from Nassau on the sloop *Only Son*, having departed on the same day as Hall set out for Green Turtle Cay. His company stopped first at Hatchet Bay, a small settlement in the north near to Gregory Town. They had planned to collect a passenger and then sail on to Governor's Harbour, where Carleton was scheduled to hold court. However, at Hatchet Bay, his landing boat was met by a barrage of stones launched by residents from the shore. The intrepid magistrate and his party dodged their way through the missiles and managed to reach land. On the shore, they pleaded with the community for cooperation, but to no avail. The residents assured Carleton that they had nothing against him personally, but they feared the introduction of cholera.[296] They prevented him from leaving the immediate vicinity of his landing and after lingering in the area for an hour he gave up and departed for Governor's Harbour. *Only Son* arrived there after dark and Carleton and his party were treated to an even more hostile reception. A shower of stones, probably flung with accuracy to purposely miss heads, splashed all around the boat as they rowed ashore. In the magistrate's scarcely believable account of derring-do, the following report was published.

'On jumping out of the boat, a scuffle ensued. Mr. C. collared one of the ringleaders, [a Mr W. A. Dean], pulled him into the boat and ordered two of the crew to take him at once on board the vessel.' Carleton then somehow calmly 'walked through a half-frantic mob that were brandishing sticks and bludgeons over their heads in all directions'. One of the rioters threatened to bash the magistrate in the head but Carleton struck the man's arm and the weapon was dropped. He went on to singlehandedly disarm a number of people in the crowd, having 'succeeded in wrenching several guns, sticks, and other weapons from the rioters'. His heroic actions in the service of Her Majesty continued when he saw that 'several parties were endeavoring to rescue the prisoner, in doing which they severely maltreated the party who had charge of him'. Carleton grabbed hold of the prisoner himself and saw to it that he was secured on board the *Only Son*, where the party withdrew for the night.

The following morning, Carleton again faced the same fearful and angry residents. Police constables were on the scene and the magistrate entreated, cautioned and then begged them for help, but they refused to lift a finger. They replied that 'they were not offending against the laws, but only protecting their lives from cholera'.

Community leaders countered the magistrate's threats with a warning of their own. Carleton was told that should cholera break out in their community, 'as was now inevitable, seeing that he and his party had landed', he would never leave the island alive. It was enough to make the magistrate beat a hasty retreat back to Nassau, and on arrival he made a beeline for Government House. His breathless report animated the chief executive and Gregory called an emergency meeting of the Executive Council.

The governor-in-council resolved to send troops to Eleuthera to restore order and to put down what it framed as an insurrection. Captain Ninian Craig, commander of the 1st West India Regiment, was summoned for the assignment and a proclamation was published announcing the action. It called the residents' mortal fear of cholera a sham and said that it was being invoked as a mere 'pretext' for disobedience. The Proclamation declared as follows.

> Whereas, authentic information has this day been received, to the effect that a considerable number of persons resident

at Hatchet Bay and Governors Harbour, in the island of Eleuthera, have conspired to prevent all intercourse with the Seat of Government, under the pretext of warding off the epidemic, which has lately unhappily prevailed in other districts of the colony, and have proceeded to various acts of lawless violence, that's endangering the public peace and the lives of her Majesty's subjects; and whereas it has become necessary to take immediate measures to put an end to the state of things, and to restore the dominion of the Law;

Now therefore I do hereby proclaim to all Her Majesty's Subjects in Eleuthera and other islands under this Government my determination forthwith to extinguish this disloyal and turbulent propensity on the part of certain portion of the people, and I do hereby accordingly make known that, acting under the advice of Her Majesty's Council, I have called upon the Military Authorities to aid and assist the Civil Power in restoring order in all those Settlements where unhappily these disaffected proceeding have taken place, and I do hereby earnestly call upon all magistrates and Public Officers, and upon all well-affected subjects of Her Majesty, to be aiding and assisting the Civil and Military Authorities in restoring and bringing the misguided population of certain of the Out Islands of this Government to a more correct perception of the criminality of their proceedings. Given under my hand at Government House, Nassau, this 27th Day of November 1852, John Gregory. By His Excellency's Command, C R Nesbitt, Colonial Secretary. God save the Queen![297]

The assignment to Eleuthera gave the West India Regiment an actual military mission, which would have come as a welcome relief from the soldiers' routine of patrols and ceremonies, and, most of all, their late confinement to barracks. The rank-and-file had been confined at the height of the epidemic to keep them safe from the disease, but the move had badly backfired. Cholera broke out in the barracks and many cases proved fatal. Confined to quarters where comrades (who remained nameless in the press) still fell ill and died had them living in terror.

Two or three months after the epidemic was over, Kirkwood traced the Regiment's outbreak to the garrison's water supply. Decades would pass before he was sufficiently comfortable to share this insight. At the time of the outbreak of this disease that no one seemed to understand, confinement appeared tantamount to a death sentence. Men were undoubtedly glad to step forward when Captain Craig called up a company of sixty of them for a mission to Eleuthera. On Monday, December 1, the detachment sailed to Governor's Harbour in the *Pedraza*, a chartered American brigantine. Dr Gavin, not to be left out of the action, volunteered to accompany the force to lend his expertise and to help bring calm.

A group that included Captain Craig and twenty-five of his soldiers, along with Police Magistrate MacCarthy, Carleton, Deputy Assistant Commander Coxworthy and Dr Gavin, were landed at Crosskill Hills near Gregory Town. From there, they marched the five miles to Hatchet Bay while the brig sailed to the settlement.

As the *Pedraza* approached Hatchet Bay, a rowboat came out to meet it, with its occupants waving them off. But when the rowers spied troops aboard, they reversed course and returned to land, only to find their village under occupation by twenty-five soldiers.

At 2 p.m. that afternoon, MacCarthy read the governor's proclamation to the gathered residents and explained to them what it meant. Gavin then addressed the crowd and told them what measures they could take in the event that cholera were to break out. Captain Craig had the five men named as the ringleaders of the opposition rounded up and taken prisoner. The party then sailed to Governor's Harbour, where the performance was repeated. Gavin formed a local Board of Health there and tutored its members on 'the best means of preventing the outbreak of cholera'. MacCarthy, Captain Craig, Coxworthy and Carleton then rode with a Reverend Williams and Mr Moss, the public schoolmaster to Palmetto Point. There, in the chapel, the Proclamation reading and health address by Dr Gavin was again repeated. The reverend then treated the party to island hospitality, with a 'substantial dinner' in the adjoining house. They returned to Governor's Harbour that very evening with the intention of sailing to Gregory Town, but at sunrise the winds refused to cooperate. It was decided that the troops were no longer needed and on December 4, rather than proceeding to Gregory Town, the *Pedraza* departed Eleuthera, leaving MacCarthy and Gavin behind. Of the other settlements they visited, it was noted that at Spanish Wells, MacCarthy and Gavin again received a hostile reception.[298]

While the detachment of troops was away, authorities condemned the barracks in New Providence as unfit for habitation and moved the remainder of the garrison.[299] The report on the mission implicated various local officials in the forming of an illegal blockade. The Council considered bringing formal charges but, in the end, the government limited its response to rebukes and reprimands. William Cash was forced to resign as a justice of the peace and Thomas Petty, a shopkeeper in Tarpum Bay, had his commission as a justice of the peace suspended.[300]

However, there was scarcely time or capacity for the government to dwell on the difficulties with its officials in Eleuthera as a new crisis arose immediately upon the return of the troops. On December 5, when the detachment sailed back to Nassau, they met an eye-popping sight in the harbour. An unfamiliar vessel lay at anchor in the port. It was the *Ovando* and she was ablaze.

# 6

## Not a Haven of Grace

The *Ovando* was an immigrant vessel that ended up in New Providence, where she met an untimely end, in the middle of the cholera epidemic.

Regardless of her Spanish name, she was an American barque. On September 29, she was one of a trio of vessels at the docks of Le Havre (along with the *Howard* and the *Tennessee*) loading up for the journey to New York.[301] When her provisions and her cargo of champagne were safely stowed, 139 German and 10 French emigrants boarded. They had paid for a no-frills passage and so they brought their own food. Rough weather delayed their departure, but on October 9, they set out for America.

Emigration was a venture for the stout of mind and body. Criminal enterprises and bad actors hovered like vultures and those that made it onto a vessel had to brave 'ship fever' and other diseases. In addition, the threat of hunger from failure to bring on sufficient food was ever-present.

The passengers aboard the *Ovando* were among the nearly 12

million who abandoned Europe for the United States in the latter half of the nineteenth century.[302] From 1845 to 1849, famine in Ireland triggered an exodus of more than a million. They were typically destitute, or nearly so, and many were ill even before they boarded a disease-ridden ship, where numbers were lost on the ocean crossing.[303] German emigration swelled to 200,000 a year during the same period, but Germans were usually literate and skilled, and so more welcomed.

In 1517, the king of France had a grand harbour built at Le Havre, a city on the north-east coast of France, which he named Havre-de-Grâce, literally 'Haven of Grace'. Over the years it was fortified and improved to such a degree that it was one of the main departure points for both French and German emigrants for the six- to ten-week ocean-crossing voyage.[304] Those bound for New Orleans had to negotiate the North-East Providence Channel of The Bahamas, where many, like the *William and Mary*, foundered.[305] Vessels like the *Ovando* that were headed to New York never came anywhere near the treacherous waters of The Bahamas. So, on Thursday, December 2, 1852, when the *Ovando* sailed into Nassau Harbour and her captain told the port health officer that they had set out from Havre-de-Grâce for New York, he was met with a confused stare.

The journey from Le Havre was benign at the beginning. Things began to go badly towards the end of the third week at sea when, on October 28, the *Ovando* sprang a leak. It was bad enough that the pumps had to be run non-stop, but now, in this condition, they ran into a storm. For forty-eight hours, wind and waves battered the ship and drove her miles south of course. So damaged was the *Ovando* that she could maintain no direction other than a south-westerly heading.[306] The situation worsened when one of her overworked pumps gave out, causing the water sloshing around inside her hull to rise to a level of several feet.

For the whole month of November, the hobbled, leaking vessel limped south-west. Food supplies were dwindling and desperation was mounting when, by a stroke of luck, it encountered the brig *Edinburgh*, sailing to Demerara (now part of Guyana). Her generous master gave Captain Higgins a barrel of flour and four barrels of potatoes, to be rationed among the hungry emigrants. It was in this sorry state that on December 2, the *Ovando* made it to New Providence.

The unexpected arrival of over 100 emigrants aboard a potentially disease-ridden ship would have been an unwelcome sight to the authorities in Nassau at any time. In the midst of the prevailing cholera epidemic, it came as a doubly unpleasant surprise. Food stocks on the island were already precarious. The market was disrupted and the limitations on the importation of fruits and vegetables imposed in September were still in place.[307] The emigrants were placed in quarantine on board the ship. Captain Higgins alone was permitted to land, and only because he needed to purchase provisions and organise repairs.

On December 6, four days into quarantine, the *Ovando* caught fire. The *Royal Gazette* described how the disaster unfolded.

> Smoke was discovered from her fore hatch at about 9 o'clock in the morning and the alarm having been immediately given, many boats filled with people and buckets were

> alongside, two engines were soon there, and every effort made to extinguish the fire, and at one time it was thought it was under control, but when the ship changed her position with the change of the tide, the fire burst out of her main and after hatches with increased violence; all hope of saving the ship was then abandoned.[308]

The first mate nearly lost his life trying to save luggage when smoke inhalation knocked him unconscious. He was dragged off the ship and revived on shore. The emigrants escaped unharmed but more than half of them got away with nothing more than the clothes on their backs. One life was lost – that of Jack Moxey, a young wrecker who twice dove and snatched items from the hull, but drowned on his third attempt.[309] The forlorn remains of the *Ovando* floated in the harbour for two days, until 1:00 p.m. on December 8, when the Royal Artillery scuttled her with twenty-one rounds fired into the hull from a six-pound gun.[310] A few days later, the merchant A. T. Holmes had quarts of salvaged champagne on sale at $10 a dozen.[311]

The suddenly homeless and penniless emigrants huddled on the wharf and then wandered about the town in shock. They were blamed for starting the fire, attributed to their habit of smoking below-decks. Governor Gregory guessed by the quality of the clothes they wore that they had not always been poor, but rather, until this moment of sudden destitution, were 'people of some little property'.

While the detachment of troops was in Eleuthera, the authorities had condemned the Fort Nassau Barracks as unfit for habitation and moved the garrison.[312] Located where the British Colonial Hilton Hotel stands today, at 1 Bay Street, the place was in rough shape even before the cholera outbreak among the troops emptied the place. The garrison had moved there from Fort Charlotte some sixteen years earlier as an escape from the mists that caused so much yellow fever. Fort Nassau was perceived as a healthier location. Governor Gregory suggested that its waterfront location was almost pretty, with its three 'well-ventilated ranges of barracks (two for the men and one for the officers)'.[313] The now-empty barracks at Fort Nassau was the only place on the island that could immediately house together all of the survivors of the *Ovando*. The place was hastily prepared for their reception.[314]

Never mind the fact that the latrines were limited in number and that there was nowhere to bathe, the *Ovando* survivors were grateful for the roof over their heads and water to drink, even though it was brackish. The recent history of the place was one cause for alarm over their housing at that location. A least one citizen came out publicly with another concern: the cost to the colony. In a letter to the editor of the *Guardian*, he lamented that 'the public and private benevolence of the Colony is liable to frequent and large appeals' that it was unable to satisfy. He urged the government to create a 'regular establishment of a house of refuge for shipwrecked and other distrest [*sic*] persons who are driven by disasters at sea to the principal port of this dangerous coast'.[315]

To help with the immediate need at hand, the governor activated the colony's diplomats. The French vice-consul visited the barracks and promised to provide for those emigrants under his jurisdiction. Care of the Germans proved to be a little more complicated. Only in July had Her Imperial Majesty approved the appointment of Robert A. Thomson to be Nassau's consul to the Free Hanseatic City of Hamburg,[316] Germania was then still a collection of city-states and not yet a single nation. When Ambassador Thomson visited the barracks, he found that none of the stranded emigrants were from his jurisdiction. He confessed to the governor that, as much as he wanted to help, in his official capacity there was very little that he could do.

After only three days of the emigrants being crammed into the barracks, the place was a pigsty. On the evening of December 9, the inevitable occurred. Joseph Bersch, a twenty-one-year-old emigrant, developed severe watery diarrhoea and died before sunrise. In the morning, as his body was removed, authorities rushed to clean and ventilate the place. Kirkwood examined everyone and, finding no one else to be ill, ordered buckets so that the visitors could take their first bath in months. He recommended their diet be upgraded to something more than their fare of biscuit and salted food. The Board of Health seconded Kirkwood's recommendation and the governor saw to it that they got 'good bread and fresh meat'.[317]

The belated attention to sanitation and nutrition could not protect the visitors from the contaminated well in the barracks yard. Its water, which had already sickened many soldiers, began doing the same to the emigrants. As they fell ill, Kirkwood had them removed to a cholera ward that he set up nearby. Rose Micklewhite, the garrison's experienced and treasured nurse, was placed in charge of the ward. A language barrier made communication difficult. Only one person in the entire group spoke English, a Monsieur Fogt. He proved to be a godsend, as he happened to be energetic, trilingual and happy to help.

The outbreak of cholera among the emigrants added urgency to the government's planning for their evacuation. It hired the *Pedraza* to take the stranded émigrés to the United States. In preparation, the ship's storage bays were replaced with berths, and a broad stairway that led from the main hatchway into the hold was built. The departure date was set for Tuesday, December 14. Dr Chipman hosted a St Andrew's Society fundraiser at his home to help with their sendoff. The £30 collected was given to Ambassador Thomson to buy and distribute whatever could be obtained with the money.[318]

Captain Higgins published a card of thanks in the press once arrangements were in hand for the way in which his passengers were to be moved out. He thanked the governor, the officers of the ordnance and Captain Craig for placing sentries at the warehouse which held what luggage and cargo they had been able to save. He also thanked Captain Scott, the fire brigade and the officers of the vessels in port, as well as the members of the general public who had pitched in to fight the fire on his ship.[319] On December 12, their final Sunday in the colony, the emigrants were treated to a very Bahamian style of hospitality. They were taken to church.

Zion Baptist Church sits on the corner of East and Shirley Streets. It opened in 1835 on property purchased from a shopkeeper named Robert Bell. When, in 1840, the Reverend Henry Capern came out from England to become the pastor, he found it (and Bethel Baptist Church on Meeting Street) in a sorry state. The London Baptist Missionary Society that sent Capern regarded Zion, together with Bethel, as one church.[320] Capern was credited with restoring both structures and their dwindling and dispersed congregations.[321] Zion Baptist Church had not yet been transformed 'to one of the prettiest buildings in town, with its columned portico in front and the interior remodeled with galleries on three sides'.

In the 1850s, the church was more like a great big barn.[322] The Honourable John S. George, the House of Assembly representative for Exuma who was also a deacon at Zion, treated the emigrants to a warm welcome at his church. Deacon George, a close associate of Reverend Capern, happened to be fluent in German. He conducted the service for the one hundred-plus visitors entirely in their language: the lessons, the prayers, hymns and sermon.[323] A reporter with a keen eye who attended the service picked out the different denominations of the faith among the emigrants by their behaviour at worship. Lutherans and Catholics, he noted, bowed at the mention of the name of Jesus Christ, while Calvinists and Baptists did not. He was moved by their singing, which, even in a tongue he could not understand, was such a choral treat that he was moved to write, 'may we one day hear the several sections of the Church of Christ in Nassau blending their voices in the praises of their Redeemer as sweetly and harmoniously as these foreigners'.[324]

Two days after the worship service, on the very morning they were to leave the barracks, cholera struck down fourteen-year-old Margaretta Palm. She was said to have been 'fine, sprightly and robust' until 1 a.m., when she fell suddenly and violently ill, dying five hours later. Under the cloud of her death, the emigrants embarked the *Pedraza.* They left ten behind: three on the cholera ward, and in the barracks a husband, a brother-in-law and five children waited for their relations to recover.

In an ominous and disastrous lapse, Joseph Schneider, a ten-year-old boy with active cholera, was taken aboard the *Pedraza.* His illness went undetected just long enough for him to contaminate the food and water on board before he died.[325] Final preparations to sail were in progress when Joseph's shrivelled corpse was carried off.[326] At the last minute a letter arrived from Governor Gregory to Monsieur Fogt. It read as follows.

> The Governor is unwilling that you should leave the Bahama Islands without receiving from the Executive Government an expression of its high sense of your valuable services in cooperating with the local authorities to relieve the unfortunate passengers of the 'Ovando' from the dreadful state of distress into which 150 human beings were suddenly thrown by the lamentable loss of the ship by fire, and by the consequent destruction of their property.
>
> The great majority of your fellow passengers being unable to speak any other language but German, the task of providing for the comfort, and more especially of attending to the more urgent wants of those who were unhappily attacked by the local epidemic, was one of some difficulty in a place where very few persons understood their language.
>
> From the concurrent testimony of the Board of Health and of the medical attendant, it appears that your personal

> exertions in constantly interpreting for the emigrants, and in various other ways cooperating with the local authorities, have been eminently useful, and he deems it to be an act of justice on your departure from the colony thus to record his sense of your conduct, believing it to have been highly honorable to your character for active humanity towards your fellow passengers in this their day of almost unparalleled misfortune. I have, &c. C R Nesbitt, Colonial Secretary. 15 December 1852.

The *Pedraza* set sail, bound not for New York but for Charleston. It was not long out of Nassau when cholera broke out on board and during the week-long voyage several more emigrants died. On December 22, when the *Pedraza* sailed into Charleston Harbour, eleven emigrants were very sick and one died just as the vessel dropped anchor.[327]

The Charleston authorities had been forewarned about inbound immigrants and began to make preparations for their quarantine. Their fate was placed in the hands of Charleston native Dr Thomas Young Simons (1797–1857), the long-standing port physician. The fifty-five-year-old graduate of the University of Edinburgh was a highly respected member of the community and he had public health credentials.[328] In 1839, as chairman of the Board of Health, he had published a short but authoritative report on yellow fever in the area.[329] His plan was to have the emigrants quarantined on Morris Island, an 840-acre island just south of Charleston's main port. Today it is uninhabited but in the 1850s it was a retreat for the well-to-do and, during the Civil

War, the site of a heralded battle. A lazaretto (quarantine station for maritime travellers) had been built on the island in the 1830s but it had been seldom used. Authorities had it hastily prepared for inmates and, for extra space, borrowed the summer homes of a Mr Bird and Captain Vincent.

Simons waited until Christmas Day, when Morris Island was ready, before he boarded the *Pedraza*. He immediately sent forty of the immigrants to the island, with the majority going to the loaned residences. Three days later, the remaining immigrants were given blankets and 'the best bread, beef, and other necessary comforts and allowed to join their fellows on the Island'.[330] Four of those taken to the lazaretto were almost dead on arrival. One succumbed on admission and the other three died in the following days.

On December 29, President J. D. Yates of the German Friendly Society of South Carolina reported that 'an application has been made asking what aid the Society would grant to the Emigrants just arrived on our shore in distress'. The plea came from Rudolph Anger, likely one of the emigrants. The Society referred it to its committee of relief to 'enquire strictly, whether they come under our rules and if so, they be authorized to extend such aid as they may deem necessary'. Up to $200 was allocated by the committee for this purpose.[331]

Despite the mortalities and all that preceded his involvement, Simons opined that the emigrants did not have cholera but some other disease. They were sick, he said, because of poor ventilation and bad clothing, made worse by the emotional distress of sudden destitution. His expertise in yellow fever was well established and his experience with cholera was about to grow. Cholera, which had not been seen in Charleston since 1836, broke out there while the emigrants were in quarantine and killed forty-nine residents over the holiday.[332] Three of those were German-born adults: August Sharlock, Nohlert and J. D. Habenitch. They may have been among those emigrants who died on Morris Island. The Charleston outbreak ended in February 1853 with a toll of eighty-five dead.[333]

Monsieur Fogt, the trilingual Frenchman, wrote back to Governor Gregory from Charleston, thanking him for the expression of esteem and praising the people of Nassau for their hospitality. He revealed that in addition to the five of his fellow passengers that died on the way to Charleston from Nassau, another seven were lost during quarantine.[334] Theodore Strempel, a fellow emigrant, also sent a heartfelt thank-you to the people of Nassau, 'on behalf of his fellow passengers'. Ambassador Thomson translated his letter from German and forwarded it to the governor.[335]

On Christmas Eve, one of the two migrants who remained on the cholera ward in Nassau died. Cholera also claimed the life of Nurse Rose Micklewhite. She fell a 'sacrifice to the disease', likely a result of her drinking from the contaminated well, as the transmission of cholera from patient to caregiver was a rare occurrence.[336] On New Year's Eve, Captain Higgins and the remaining emigrants boarded the RMS *Conway*, bound for Savannah, Georgia, finally escaping the place that proved to be anything but a haven of grace.[337]

On January 5, the *Ovando* survivors in America were released from quarantine on Morris Island. The mayor authorised a contribution of $300 from the city treasury for relief and transportation for those still intent on getting to New York.[338] The survivors dispersed, becoming members of the French and German diaspora whose descendants helped to make America a mighty nation.

# 7

## Salus Populi Suprema Lex

In the New Year, 1853, the wheels of normal commerce began turning again in the capital and the government got back to its regular business. Election campaigning resumed for House of Assembly representatives for districts in New Providence and for Eleuthera and Long Island.[339] Duncome entered the race as a candidate for the Town District of New Providence. Farre, even though 'anxious and exhausted' from the strain of superintending the Cholera Hospital, contested the seat for the Western District of New Providence.[340]

Duncome was successful and became the Member-elect for his district, along with T. M. Matthew, R. Bell and Stephen Dillet. He thanked his supporters and promised that, 'as a Bahamian, when he took his seat in the new House of Assembly, he would do his utmost to merit their continued confidence and support'. The nervous Henry Farre was defeated.[341]

Days after Duncome's successful election, on January 11, the Reverend Dr Strachan, rector of Christ Church, called the Sunday

School superintendent and his teachers to a meeting. Cholera had killed one of their number and caused the cancellation of the church's popular annual bazaar, an important fundraiser. Duncome's presence along with the other attendees demonstrated that the general fear of social gatherings was rapidly dissipating. He tried to boost his team's morale, assuring them that they would regroup and resume the school and the bazaar in the coming months.[342] It was a promise that he fulfilled.[343]

Residents may have hoped that cholera had left Nassau for good with the departure of the last of the refugees from the *Ovando*, but the disease was still around. In fact, New Providence experienced a smaller second wave. In early January, this caused the Board of Health to urge residents to visit one of the six established depots to get their supply of medicines. It republished the 'premonitory symptoms' of the disease and warned that these should be taken seriously and immediately treated. As the Board correctly put it, 'whenever Asiatic cholera is epidemic, the very slightest degree of looseness of the bowels ought to be regarded and treated as the commence [*sic*] of the disease'. It stuck to the fallacy that one could prevent mild diarrhoea from becoming cholera if people started treatment at the first sign of stomach trouble. And the Board emphasised that the stimulants and potions it recommended and had supplied to the house-to-house visitors were the only ones to be employed. It scolded that many people had died unnecessarily from them 'placing a vain and most dangerous confidence in remedies of their own selection, or of their own compounding'.[344]

No doubt, the Board of Health was talking primarily to the

10,000-odd Black people who had been enslaved just fourteen years earlier. Its manner of superiority and presumed monopoly on health information demonstrated how colonial rulers in the post-Emancipation period found in healthcare a new avenue for power displays.[345]

Regardless of whether one trusted or avoided the Board's recommendations, there was no way to sugarcoat the terrifying implication that a grumbling stomach and a little diarrhoea could mean that you might be dead before the day was out.

❦ ❦ ❦

While the public grappled with the loss of so many loved ones, the keepers of the public purse fretted over the flood of disaster-related bills. On January 3, at the Executive Council's first meeting of the year, it studied a bill that came in from Bimini for the payment of the labourers who had cleaned roads by order of the Board of Health. It was only for £13.19s, but the governor cut it down to £6.19s.7d on the basis that Bimini labourers should be paid the same 50 cents per day as workers in Nassau received. The second bill examined by the Council at that meeting was for a whopping £350 from Dr Kirkwood. It was for medicines he had supplied in New Providence during the first months of the epidemic.[346] The governor referred it to the House of Assembly and the House referred it to a select committee.

The Board of Health continued to harry the Council for resources, in part to expand the usefulness of the house-to-house visitors. As they moved through the community, the visitors were encountering numerous persons who may have been cholera-free, but were regardless in desperate need of help. Some were malnourished, others were sick and still others were clearly destined to be so. Merely checking to see whether anyone in the house had cholera and offering opium did them no good. The stories they brought back to the Board from their rounds, of visiting people with barely enough to eat, shocked the Board into asking the government to make some provisions for them. It called for the employment of a special relieving officer for the 'outdoor poor'. It also asked for the appointment of two additional constables to enforce sanitary regulations. The governor-in-council referred the request for a special relieving officer to the commissioners of the New Providence Asylum and dismissed the other.[347]

On January 17, two weeks after entertaining the Board's earlier requests, the Executive Council reconvened with the verdict of the commissioners of the Asylum in hand. The commissioners were sympathetic to the Council's reluctance to expand the public expenditure and advised that they saw no need for a special relieving officer for the poor.[348] However, the Council now had a new request from Gavin – a list of 'queries' for public information and reflection, which he wanted printed and distributed. The Council ruled the communication a private pursuit.

Medical Inspector Gavin became frustrated by the Council's denial of all recent requests from himself and the Board. On the heels of this setback came word that Chipman, Duncome and Kirkwood were abandoning the districts created by the Board of Health. Henceforth, they would be going wherever they were called and they would charge their usual fee for service. The loss of their cooperation with the Board further distanced and diminished the influence of the inspector.

Gavin sensed that the denial of his requests was not simply due to a lack of funds. Kirkwood was getting paid. His latest bill of £101.5s, for medicines that he had sent to the out islands, was favorably considered. The governor sought the doctor's assurance that the supplies were being billed at the same rate paid by the Public Dispensary. Kirkwood gave his word, and on January 17, his invoice was approved for immediate payment.[349] At the same time, the Council began rolling back the funding and powers of the Board of Health. It took aim first at Gavin's signature programme: house-to-house visitation.

As cholera cases continued to fall off in New Providence, the Council judged the expense of house-to-house visitation no longer necessary. It let some visitors go and told those remaining to stick to their job of attention to cholera only. It did not want to even hear about any other needs and told the visitors that they were to cease bringing cases of 'mere destitution' to the attention of the Board of Health.[350]

The inspector had been pushed as far as he could go, and was at the point of blowing up at the leadership, as he had done in spectacular fashion in his *Sanitary Ramblings*. Already, he had anonymously published a piece that had strongly criticised the government's response to the epidemic.[351] The governor had seen it and dismissed it as coming from some curmudgeon in the community who had no clue. However, a few days after the Council cut back the house-to-house visitors programme, Gregory was tipped off that Gavin was in fact the author of the critique.

He confronted Gavin, who stood there tight-lipped, refusing to confirm or deny authorship. Gregory took this as an admission of guilt and fired him on the spot. Chief Justice Lees was appointed as the new chairman of the Board of Health and the house-to-house visitors were given notice that they would all be let go in February.

Gavin told his colleagues that he had resigned and began preparations to leave town. He gave the impression that he would go quietly. He paid a courtesy call on the trustees of the Nassau Public Library and presented a gift of pamphlets published by London's General Board of Health, including two that he had authored.[352] On Saturday, January 29, the Board of Health held a farewell dinner in his honour. Some of the attendees, like his medical colleagues, were probably there with mixed feelings. Others were unquestionably sad to see him leaving. Gavin had made friends in the colony; Captain Craig, Justice Carleton and John Bacon, the American vice-consul, came to show their support. So too did Reverend Duncome, the sitting chairman of the Harbour Island Board of Health. Notably absent from the event were the governor, the colonial secretary and Justice Lees.

When the Executive Council met days after the dinner, on February 2, the medical inspector never came up for discussion. It was relieved to find that for the first time in weeks, no requests from the Board of Health had come in, other than a call for an additional £200 in funding. The Council also entertained other cholera-related expenses. A bill came from Mr Robert Bell on Harbour Island to the amount of £2.5s.10d for providing nurses with housing. Another came from Mr W. Barker for his services as acting nurse at Hope Town and Little Guana Cay. He sought remuneration at 'whatever the scale is for nurses'.[353] Mr Bullard in George Town, Exuma requested payment for supplies that he had provided and Mr Mardenbough, the receiver (and future police magistrate) for Harbour Island, submitted that island's Board of Health cholera-related expenses, which amounted to over £300.[354] The Council clamped down. It cancelled the authority of all colonial receivers to advance any more money for cholera-related expenses.

On February 5, 1853, seven days after the banquet held in his honour, Gavin dropped a bombshell in *The Nassau Guardian*: a polemic in which he insulted practically everyone with whom he had worked, from the governor down to the humble house-to-house foot soldiers.[355] Gavin quoted Cicero, the great Roman statesman: '*Salus populi suprema lex esto*' ('The health of the people is the supreme law'). Lawyers and statesmen have upheld this dictum for at least 2,000 years and Gavin slammed the governor for failing to follow this ancient rule. He held forth that Governor Gregory had blocked everything that he had tried to do to protect the colony from cholera, with the exception of the house-to-house visitation programme. 'It is unnecessary for me to enter upon the obstructive course pursued in regard to nearly all the other measures which were recommended', wrote the inspector. In his view, the government had not worked hard enough to contain the epidemic. His colleagues had not cooperated with the Board of Health, and when he had asked for the Council to compel them to do so, he had been 'rebuffed' by the governor. This, he stated, had been the final straw that had caused his resignation.

Gavin placed great weight on the system of house-to-house visitation, which the government terminated on January 29. He published a complex table of statistics that he claimed contained irrefutable proof of the lifesaving effectiveness of the programme. Discovering evidence of lifesaving benefit in the inspector's web of statistics could be likened to finding faces in clouds. It could be seen that the programme had provided temporary employment for eight persons and it is imagined that some who were visited welcomed the attention, but that was about it. Some residents would have experienced visitation as a programme of forced observation by outsiders, and this during a time of great personal and family stress.

The statistics bear witness to the diligence of the visitors. In their first week, over the course of 43 home visits, they discovered 213 cases and 20 persons who had died of cholera. None of them had seen a doctor, visited the Dispensary or asked for any help. In total, they discovered 1,800 persons with cholera. Of those, 190 were severely or critically ill when found, and the visitors endured the ordeal of watching 87 people die.

Gavin, perhaps appreciating that extraordinary intelligence was required to properly interpret his statistics, sought to strengthen his case of the benefit of his programme with testimonials from his colleagues. He had contacted each of them before dropping his bombshell, and now he trotted out their responses for the public.[356]

Chipman wrote, 'While you were absent in the infected Islands of Harbour Island and Eleuthera, I had an opportunity of seeing more completely the effects of house-to-house visitation, having been appointed by you to receive the reports of the Visitors. This opportunity only tended to affirm the high estimate, which I had previously formed of this plan of operation.' Kirkwood was measured and wary in his answer to Gavin's request for commentary, as if he could see the hook in the bait. He responded by first repeating Gavin's obviously leading question: 'Having been asked to state my opinion of the value of an efficient system of house-to-house visitation in relation to the prevention of the spread of cholera…' Kirkwood pointed out that unpaid visitors had attended the poor prior to Gavin's arrival, and that they had done 'incalculable good'. Only then did he acknowledge that paid visitors under Gavin's direction were more effective. Even then, he pointed out that this was so because they were organised, supervised and paid. Only after this preface did the wise physician allow, 'I have no hesitation in stating that the system of house-to-house visitation is the only one on which I would on any future occasion rely for the prevention of the spread of epidemic cholera.' Home visitation was even more important in Nassau, he continued, where the population 'consists of the most part of Africans and native blacks, whose ignorance, apathy and prejudices caused them to abstain from making any application at the local dispensaries for medicines until all aid was too late, and in consequence, numbers died without having received any medicines or medical aid whatever.'

Gavin, with his colleagues' endorsements safely in hand, informed the public that his visitation system would have been more effective had the visitors been more intelligent and the supervising doctors properly qualified. He wrote the following.

> I do not pretend for a moment that it was as sufficiently carried out as the visitation in the districts of London which I had charge of in 1849, but, considering that the persons employed here as Visitors were of an humble class in society, and (with the exception of one or two) were not of more than a very ordinary degree of intelligence, whereas the parties employed in London were educated professional men and advanced students of medicine, [paid] at from four to six guineas per week, and were constantly supervised by Inspectors specially qualified in the work of prevention.

Gavin tried to end his letter with a measure of grace, but even this he spoiled with a slur. He thanked his colleagues for their assistance with his programme and then slapped them with the statement that there would have been fewer widows and orphans in the colony had they been more cooperative with the Board of Health.

Having blasted all of the socially and professionally connected men who ran the colony, Gavin had no intention of waiting around in Nassau for consequences. On February 8, he boarded the RMS *Conway* and departed.[357]

Gavin's tirade was met with official silence. On Tuesday, February 22, the governor addressed newly elected parliamentarians and members of the Legislative Council at the opening of the 1853 session of the House of Assembly. He began as follows.

> The period at which I have called you together for the purpose of Legislation, is one which will occupy a space painfully remarkable in the history of the Bahamas. These

> islands, enjoying the most salubrious climate of the West Indies, have so long been blessed with an exemption from any fatal epidemic that the awful pestilence which has just swept over us with almost unexampled severity and carried to their graves so large a portion of our population came upon the colony as unexpected as the Tornado of 1850.[358]

Gregory was not being completely truthful when he claimed that cholera had caught the colony by surprise. The Colonial Office had appointed Gavin and the other inspectors specifically because it anticipated cholera would reach its West Indies colonies. Gregory was aware of the progress of the pandemic, its ravages in Jamaica and of Gavin's presence in Trinidad long before The Bahamas was hit.

He was on safer ground in defending the actions of his administration after the epidemic arrived. 'I am prepared to say that all was done which could be done to limit the progress of so fatal an epidemic; but this I can safely say, that so far as the existing law of the colony enabled the executive government to go, nothing was left undone that could reasonably be regarded as necessary or as really useful.' Even here, Gregory was hedging. The government response to the epidemic was limited not so much by the law as by the willingness of the government to pay for services. Gregory also touted his administration's support of the house-to-house visitation programme and again, without naming Gavin, refuted the inspector's most damning allegation.

> [T]he Executive Government cannot justly be accused of 'pursuing an obstructive course' when its sanction was readily

> given (utterly regardless of expense) to a system which the highest professional opinions in the colony have subsequently pronounced to be the *only* one to be relied upon for the prevention of the spread of Epidemic Cholera.

Gregory admitted that the sanitary and quarantine law of the land needed updating and then he pivoted to the colony's finances. He noted that although the epidemic had paralysed commerce in the final three months of 1852, the colony's total revenue was up over the previous year.[359] He was enthusiastic about the potential for a health tourism industry. He told the assembled legislators, 'I seized the opportunity afforded me by my recent visit to Philadelphia and New York to spread the advantages which the winter climate of The Bahamas holds out to those who are suffering from pulmonary weakness.'

The House of Assembly heard the governor's charge and committed to relooking at the quarantine law. It appointed select committees to examine the existing system 'of affording medical relief and supplying medicines to the poor' and 'to enquire into the state of the sanitary and quarantine laws of the Colony'.[360] The formation of these committees was a tacit admission that the inspector had raised legitimate concerns. As the legislators got to work, the governor waited to hear from the Colonial Office on his difficulties with the medical inspector. In the lull, it occurred to Gregory that this was an opportune time for a National Day of Thanksgiving and Prayer for the passing of the epidemic. A grand activity (or distraction), and possibly a private celebration for Gavin's departure, was conceived. He was certain that it would attract the same broad support and participation as before. The governor could never have dreamed how contentious the move would become. But he walked into a nasty spat with the pastor of Bethel Baptist Church, and how it unfolded served some insight into the workings of the colony.

❦ ❦ ❦

The Baptist denomination had the largest following in the colony. At the time of the cholera epidemic, its leadership came from the Baptist Missionary Society in England. The Reverend Henry Capern had been in the colony for thirteen years when the cholera epidemic struck. Capern was revered for having taught labourers to read and for his passion for founding schools, financed in part by funds coaxed from his parent organisation. In New Providence alone, Capern planted churches in the African villages of Gambier, Adelaide and Fox Hill.[361] During the epidemic, he worked as one of the house-to-house visitors. On Rum Cay on November 14, 1852, in the midst of the epidemic, he laid the cornerstone for a new chapel, called Zion.[362]

Bethel Baptist Church lost an eighth of its members to the epidemic.[363] No other denomination suffered nearly as great a loss. Even before the final count was known, surviving members began holding services of thanksgiving for the passage of the epidemic. Governor Gregory had a similar idea for the entire colony – a National Day of Thanksgiving and Prayer for the passing of the epidemic. In February 1853, he made his idea known, with no reason to suspect that it might be contentious. A day of prayer and humiliation had been observed at the height of the epidemic, on October 7, 1852, with general participation. Who could possibly object to now giving thanks to God for His ending of the epidemic? Gregory proposed February 17. In a praiseworthy signal of his style of governance, on February 4, he had the colonial secretary write to religious leaders asking for their feedback on the idea and the proposed date. All but one clergyman quickly responded with an indication of support.

On February 8, with an overwhelmingly positive consensus in hand, the governor drew up a proclamation. It announced that a National Day of Thanksgiving and Prayer would be observed on Thursday, February 24 in New Providence and on March 10 in the Out Islands.

> Whereas, it recently pleased the Almighty God to visit the Inhabitants of the Bahama Islands with a direful pestilence which, in the inscrutable purposes of His Providence, carried to their graves a very large proportion of the Population; And Whereas, during the prevalence of that epidemic Her Majesty's Subjects of all Religious Denominations concurred in the propriety of setting apart two days of General Fast and humiliation, and of prayers to the Throne of Mercy, for the removal of the fatal scourge; And, Whereas, it having pleased the Giver of all Good, in his infinite Mercy, to withdraw his chastening judgement, it becomes to duty of all rightly-disposed persons, to offer up praises and thanksgivings to Him in whose hands are the issues of life and death. Now, therefore, being desirous, that all Her Majesty's Subjects may

> have an opportunity of doing so simultaneously, and free from the distraction of worldly pursuits, I do hereby proclaim Thursday the seventeenth day of the present month of February, to the day on which I earnestly invite all persons whatsoever, who may be religiously and devoutly disposed to abstain from all ordinary occupations and to dedicate its hours to the solemn purposes of praise and thanksgiving for the great mercies vouchsafed to the Community'.[364]

Capern was incensed. He had meant to consult his congregation before responding to the colonial secretary's invitation, but he had missed the unspoken deadline. That the government had made the announcement without hearing from him he took as a deliberate snub. The move confirmed in his eyes the appearance that the colony's leadership held his congregation in contempt. He told the colonial secretary that as a consequence of the day being set without his having had an opportunity to respond, the Baptists would not be participating. His congregation had already held several thanksgiving services of their own, he said, and so they did not feel the need to participate in the government-organised event. It would be more godly, continued Capern, for his members to work on the Thursday, so as to give a fair day's work for pay, rather than staying at home.

Secretary Nesbitt's retort was sharp. 'His Excellency's object was to consult the Ministers of Religion – not the congregations, of all denominations; but as you deem it necessary, before letting the Governor know your own sentiments, to consult your congregation, the Governor regrets that you did not do so on

Sunday.' There was more than prejudice to Baptists missing the boat on the day of prayer. An administrative and denominational divide existed which the colonial secretary and governor had failed to see. The state-supported Anglican and Presbyterian Churches were beholden to the governor for the approval of clergy appointments, the payment of salaries and even the granting of vacation leave. The governor's suggestion to them that they participate in a day of prayer carried the force of a request, while the Baptist Church and its ministers were fully independent. Capern really did need to consult his congregation. Compounding the misunderstanding was the spot of trouble that the reverend was already having with the government over a shipment of goods.

The reverend's trouble had begun three months earlier, on November 16, when the schooner *Lelia* arrived from London via St Thomas with eight cases of goods consigned to him. The morning after its arrival, the reverend's dear friend Deacon John S. George completed the customs entry on his behalf. The whole shipment was declared to be printed books for use at the Baptist school. Deacon George could not be completely certain about the contents of every box and he claimed that he had been given the option to change the customs entry should it be found that there were more than books in the boxes.[365] He might have exercised a little more caution with the declaration had he known that the reverend's shipments had been under covert surveillance by the colony's receiver-general.

John Grant Anderson was a hawk in government whose wrong side was best avoided. He was a native son, a descendant of Loyalists, who had served in the military. In 1815, as an eighteen-year-old lieutenant with the 2nd West India Regiment, he had sailed on the *Brune* from Nassau to Georgia with a force of 300 soldiers to relieve the British who had stormed Fort Peitrie and taken the town of St Mary.[366] In 1834, he began a three-year term as the clerk of the House of Assembly, a posting that ensured his expertise in rules and procedures of the colony's over-100-year-old Parliament.[367]

In 1841, Anderson was appointed to the position of receiver-general. This job came with an *ex-officio* seat on the Executive Council and guaranteed him an intimate insight into the colony's affairs.[368] The receiver-general was responsible for collecting the 5-per-cent duty that the government assessed on everything except schoolbooks. As soon as Deacon George had completed the customs entry for the reverend's goods, Anderson intercepted the shipment and demanded that all of the boxes be opened then and there, in his presence.

The eight crates were pried open and, lo and behold, only five of them contained schoolbooks. Two contained slates and pencils. One was full of ladies' apparel – bracelets, bonnets and 'fancy goods' – along with three bottles of medicine. Anderson had everything but the books seized and called in local merchants to have them assessed. The seized items were valued at £17.15s, which amounted to an obligation of 17s.5d in duty for the government. The receiver-general immediately accused the reverend of attempting to defraud the Treasury. George leapt to Capern's defence and reiterated that a customs officer had not only given him permission to change the entry if necessary, but that he had done so 'within earshot of the receiver-general'. Anderson countered that this could never have happened. 'The normal process for clearing a shipment when one does not know or cannot remember what was being imported is to declare "Contents unknown" on the Customs entry', he returned.

The Council soon learned the reason that the receiver-general had happened to be lurking near to a junior officer when the reverend's seemingly pedestrian shipment was being cleared at the warehouse. Anderson had been watching the reverend for some time, suspicious that he had been importing goods for sale in his wife's shop under the guise of bringing in duty-free schoolbooks.

Capern asked to be allowed to pay the duty and have his goods released but the receiver-general was determined to make an example of the minister. Rather than release the goods, Anderson called for them to be put up for auction.[369] Capern appealed to the governor and, before word of the accusation of dishonesty reached his congregation, he shared details of the affair in church. Capern then informed the Baptist Missionary Society in London, which wrote to the Colonial Office on his behalf.

On November 29, Mrs Capern chimed in, appealing directly to Governor Gregory. She produced supporting correspondence from the 'benevolent Ladies' who had collected and shipped the articles from England to New Providence. They had expressly written that the items were to be sold 'to aid in our educational efforts'. She pled that the customs entry could not be completed with any accuracy in advance because neither she nor anyone else really knew what her supporters had sent. She implored the governor to intervene. He replied that he would raise the matter with his Council and would act on its advice.[370]

February rolled around, the day of prayer came and went, and the shipment had still not been released. Capern heard that tongues were wagging at Government House and that disapproving fingers in high circles were being pointed in his direction. Believing that the governor was being unfairly swayed against him and that there were important facts that might have escaped His Excellency's notice, he wrote to the commander-in-chief. He thought that the missive he had prepared was a fair and forthright explanation of what had actually transpired, but, just to be safe, he ran a draft of the letter by a wealthy and highly respected visitor.

Vere Foster (1819–1900) was famous as a philanthropist and educationalist in his day. In the 1850s, he made many visits to the United States to oversee his programme of paying for the transportation and support of Irish emigrants. On one of his trips, he made a month-long visit to New Providence. While there, he adopted the Girls' Central School, paying for an additional teacher and providing prize money for the top academic performers. He and Capern shared a passion for education and the two became fast friends. The philanthropist attended Bethel Baptist Church to hear his pal preach. He occasionally called at Capern's house and even lobbied for government support of Baptist schools.[371] Foster read a draft of the reverend's letter and gave it the thumbs-up. 'The governor needs to hear this', he said.

It was a mistake. The governor took offence at something in Capern's letter and allowed the auction to go ahead. Adding insult to injury, the law provided that half of the proceeds realised from the sale of any seized goods went personally to the governor. At this low point, Foster deserted his friend. Claiming that he was being unwillingly dragged into a matter that was not his concern, he published a disclaimer stating that he had neither sanctioned nor approved the reverend's remarks.[372]

Capern escalated his protest. He charged that the government was acting out of spite because of his refusal to support the National Day of Thanksgiving and Prayer. The colonial secretary cynically replied that 'His Excellency is at a loss to understand what connexion [*sic*] there is between the seizure of your goods and the appointment of a day for a public and general thanksgiving for the cessation of cholera.'

Word of the fracas reached the Colonial Office. The Duke of Newcastle, who had replaced Pakington at the end of 1852 as head of the Colonial Office, called on Gregory for a report. The governor's May 3 reply to the Colonial Office revealed how much the incident had blown up. The matter was now before the House of Assembly and he could only write that the affair was far too complicated to explain in the few hours available before the departure of the next mail. He asked the duke for more time to report, writing, 'I shall be prepared to furnish your Grace a full and circumstantial report upon the whole of this case, which has continued to be the subject of the most violent and unseemingly discussion in the colony for the last five months.'[373]

Capern, no doubt exhausted by the fiasco on the heels of the demanding and frightening epidemic, felt the need for a break from his pastoral work. On May 7, a body of his congregation escorted him to the waterfront, many of them openly weeping. There, he boarded the *Pedraza* to New York, headed home for the first time in more than a decade. *The Nassau Guardian* pointed to the size and conduct of the company that walked with the reverend as evidence of the 'high respect and esteem entertained for him by his members; sentiments that are participated in by the community generally'. The Reverend Dr William Maclure, who would be vacationing in Scotland, joined him aboard, as did his former friend, Vere Foster.[374]

On May 4, a few days before Capern's departure, Gregory heard at last from His Grace the Duke of Newcastle on the fracas with the fired medical inspector. The duke expressed his regret that 'the valuable services which have been rendered by Dr Gavin should have thus terminated', but he agreed that, under the circumstances, he had to be let go. The show of support made Gregory as happy as a man just given a major promotion and he dashed to set the public record straight. Before the day was out, *The Nassau Guardian* had a notice from the government that set out 'the circumstances which led to the removal of Dr. Gavin from the Board of Health, and to his being suspended from the exercise in this Island of his official functions as Medical Inspector'.[375] Penned by the colonial secretary, it contained none of the piety that would have been expected of his son, Deacon Nesbitt.[376] It pummelled Gavin, describing him as a mere public functionary who had assailed the administration, anonymously at first, in 'offensive and unjust' comments and then openly in the press on February 4. The notice informed the public that the governor had given the inspector an ultimatum, 'to disavow authorship of the obnoxious article' or be terminated. Nesbitt's notice was virtually petulant in how it took pains to let people know that the governor had fired the inspector before he quit. 'It is true that Dr Gavin did send in his resignation of the seat he held at the Board of Health', stated the notice, 'but it came too late'.

The government's version of these events was probably now of little interest to the wider community. The price for pineapples in New York was collapsing and, as the governor had predicted, pineapple-speculating farmers and shippers would now be losing money. The situation was even worse in Grand Bahama, where the crops had failed and residents were facing a risk of starvation – a problem that lingered on that island well into the next century.[377]

While Grand Bahama residents and pineapple farmers suffered, the residents of Inagua were imploring the governor for a hospital. 'We want a hospital', they pleaded, 'because the public is very suspicious of disease being landed, without any proper place to put them in'. Then, on May 3, the *William and Mary* sank while transiting the waters of the colony. The captain resurfaced in New York, where he claimed to have helplessly watched his ship sink, and to have witnessed the drowning of all who remained on board. A furore followed after the supposedly drowned passengers, who were rescued by Bahamian wreckers, revealed the truth about the cowardice of their captain.[378]

The needs of the *William and Mary* survivors, some of whom fell ill in Nassau and whose welfare was now the subject of international press attention, added to the problems on the government's plate. While this was going on, supporters of Reverend Capern launched a fundraiser, which quickly raised enough to replace the goods that were seized. This must have pricked the conscience of the government over its treatment of the beloved minister. On May 10, the House of Assembly committee that was formed to investigate the matter announced that it had completed its report. The colonial secretary, who was a member of the committee, tried to sequester the findings but it emerged that Capern and Deacon George had been exonerated.[379] Its findings returned to the government a good measure of the embarrassment that it had heaped on the Baptist leader.[380] The governor, blushing, donated his share of the auction proceeds to the Board of Education.[381]

# 8

# A Reckoning

During its early weeks, the cholera epidemic was killing an average of thirteen people a day, with a peak of twenty-eight in one twenty-four-hour period[382] – this at a time when the population of the whole colony was smaller than the total of present-day Grand Bahama. In the first nine weeks of the epidemic, New Providence lost 6.3 per cent of its population. By comparison, over a period of three years, the Covid-19 pandemic that so bloated the newspapers' obituary supplements killed just 0.3 per cent of the total population of The Bahamas. By this metric alone, the cholera epidemic was more than twenty times worse. Harbour Island's estimated 600 deaths, or 33 per cent of its residents, over the duration of the epidemic is difficult to fathom.

The Methodist Church, which reported that it 'lost some members to the Dread Disease, which raged with peculiar malignancy', managed to find a bright side. It celebrated the fact that some individuals were driven to seek out what they had to do to be saved.[383] Those followers it lost to the epidemic likely all came from the Black membership of Grants Town Wesley Methodist Church. Cholera has no natural racial preference, but in The Bahamas epidemic, its victims were overwhelmingly Black people.

Inspector Gavin asked the Nassau doctors what they estimated the mortality to be of Black residents among those they had treated. Dr Black placed the figure at 97 per cent of those with severe cholera. Kirkwood and Duncome estimated that 80–90 per cent of the Black people they had treated died, and Chipman pegged it at 80 per cent. These figures are considerably higher than the mortality at the cholera hospital, but they were counting every patient that they encountered, many of whom never got anywhere near the hospital. In fact, the doctors came across so many patients at home who were about to die that they caused the Board of Health to publish a notice that pleaded with people not to bring persons to the cholera hospital when they were deathly ill.[384]

Gavin noted that the White population seldom developed severe cholera and, when they did, they were less likely to die.[385] He found that for New Providence, for the twelve months to February 1853, there were 714 deaths from cholera and another 125 from other causes. This amounted to the loss of 8.8 per cent of the island's population of 8,159 from the cholera epidemic. He added that, 'If only the population of the affected districts were counted, then the mortality would be 18 to 23 per cent.'[386]

The disproportionate mortality of Black people to cholera was a region-wide phenomenon. The British Foreign Office estimated that Cuba lost some 46,000 enslaved people in its 1850–1854 epidemic, but only a tiny fraction of its White residents. Puerto

Rico documented that during its epidemic of 1855, Black people were three times more likely to die from the cholera than others.[387] In Barbados and in Trinidad, commentators emphasised that cholera victims were overwhelmingly poor and from the Black race.

Several explanations for the predominance of Black people among the cholera mortality statistics have been proposed. One is the presence of *Helicobacter pylori* infection, which is more prevalent among the poor.[388] This bacterium lives in the stomach and over time causes a reduction in acid secretion. Since stomach acid protects against cholera *Vibrios*, its loss increases susceptibility to cholera.

Poverty also led to malnutrition and this increased susceptibility to cholera. Farre attributed the high mortality rate of Black people to their 'reduced vitality'. He made no specific reference to their diet or nutrition during his tour at the Bain Town Cholera Hospital, but Gavin Milroy, the medical inspector to Jamaica, did. He observed that they subsisted on 'a diet unwholesome and often scanty'.[389] Pellagra, as mentioned in the first chapter, was common. More than a few persons probably had early symptoms, including pellagra-induced diarrhoea, even before cholera struck. Others were simply weakened by vitamin deficiency and less able to fight a serious illness.

The government's neglect of its Black residents contributed to their poverty. But even as the government disregarded the needs of the humble class, it bragged about all that it was doing for them. The governor trumpeted the schools opened, while admitting that they were too few and that the teachers were barely literate. Gregory showed his face at the New Providence Asylum and he highlighted the opening of the Public Dispensary, where the poor received free medical care. It made for good reporting in his despatches to England, but the government was tight-fisted with its charity. Its services were woefully underfunded and at every turn it placed strictures to access. It blocked the medical inspector's efforts to empower health officers to have a say in admissions to the Asylum. This remained firmly in the hands of the commissioners. It stopped the Board of Health from assisting the poor from the cholera emergency fund. These cold-hearted actions underscored how little the government really wanted to do. Little wonder that the fatalities from cholera came overwhelmingly from the Black population.

A clearer picture of the human cost of the epidemic can be gained by pulling back from the weekly statistics released by the Board of Health and looking at the official annual mortality figures.

The colony experienced 576 or fewer total deaths each year from 1846 through 1855, with one exception; in 1852, the number spiked to 1,656 deaths, an increase of some 1,200 over previous years (see Appendix 5). This increase, referred to by public health professionals as 'excess deaths', was caused directly or indirectly by the cholera epidemic. After the epidemic, the number fell back to fewer than 500 annually. Even a century later, in the 1950s, with a population of over 80,000 and with tuberculosis rife in the community, the colony saw nowhere near the mortality of the year cholera struck. The Bahamas was an independent nation when, in 1974, the annual mortality broke the 1,000-deaths-a-year barrier again for the first time. Only in 1995 did the mortality surpass the 1852 figure of over 1,600 deaths.[390]

Considering the awful mortality, the climb of the colony's population post-disaster at first seems counterintuitive. The population was growing at an annual rate of 0.6 per cent before the epidemic. Afterwards, the rate quadrupled to 2.9 per cent.[391] Immigration, both voluntary and involuntary, contributed to the population growth. Increased fertility may also have played a role.

The colonial government encouraged immigration. The well-heeled were invited to come and enjoy the colony's healthy climate. Labourers, who were needed for the rapidly developing salt industry, were enticed with the promise of land. The Crown offered up thousands of acres in Inagua, St Salvador, Crooked Island and Long Island, land that could yield 'millions of bushels of salt to the industry of man'. A few Englishmen already held leases and Governor Gregory suggested that Irishmen might come, and bring their families as well, if given state assistance. However, his pitch was primarily to free Black people in America because he did not think that Irish and English labourers would be able to stand the work in a tropical climate.[392] The colonial secretary echoed the governor's invitation.

> The free coloured population of the neighbouring continent of America, where they remain in a state of comparative degradation, might in this colony find, within a few days' travel by water, a climate adapted to their health, institutions encouraging the development of the mental faculties, and

> calculated to raise them in their own estimation, and enable them to exercise political, civil and social rights and privileges, and to advance themselves and children in religious knowledge, moral habits and general intelligence.[393]

The rights and privileges to which Secretary Nesbitt alluded were freedoms relative to Black people in the United States. He was not suggesting political or social equality with White residents. Still, those desirable visitors who wished to stay could be naturalised in the colony with a minimum of red tape. All that was required was for an individual 'of good character' to apply to the governor, to provide proof that they had resided in the colony for at least twelve months and to pay a small fee.

In addition to the trickle of voluntary immigrants, involuntary arrivals boosted the population. On July 28, 1860, the slave ship *Peter Mowell*, bound for Cuba, wrecked at Lanyard Cay, near Abaco. More than 200 children were among the 389 Congo Africans that were rescued and quarantined on Athol Island. In New Providence, they were housed in the military barracks, which in the wake of the cholera disaster was now back at Fort Charlotte. They remained there until distributed as indentured servants. These new arrivals were counted in the 1861 Census.

Finally, the remarkable climb in the population after the epidemic may have come in part from an increase in the birth rate. Births in the colony typically exceeded deaths by a factor of about two, so a natural increase would be anticipated. The Blue Book statistics on births are spotty for most of the years bracketing the epidemic, but the expected steady rise is evident, from 1,177 births in 1851 to 1,276 in 1856. Multiple studies have documented increases in fertility following natural disasters,[394] famine and war.[395] The magnitude of the change in The Bahamas in the wake of the cholera epidemic, if any, invites further study.

* * *

The colony's administration did not dwell on the terrible human cost of the disaster. Its main concern in the early post-epidemic months of 1853 was the financial cost to the colony. At the March 2nd meeting of the Executive Council, bills from Chipman, Duncome and Black were tabled. Each had asked to be paid the £16.16s (approximately $2,500 today) earned while they had been in the employ of the Board of Health. Clutsam billed £102.18s (equivalent to $15,000 today) for the forty-nine days from November 27 to January 14 that he had worked in Eleuthera. He tried to grease the wheels by mentioning in his cover letter that he was working on a 'Clerical Thesis on Cholera', which he was looking forward to presenting to His Excellency.[396] Wendel billed over £119 for his fifty-seven days in Harbour Island and Eneas' bill was just over £142.[397] They had earned around triple the annual salary of a typical civil servant for their epidemic work.

The governor was not happy with any of the statements of account. The fact the Out Island doctors were being paid the same £2.2s per diem as their New Providence counterparts upset him. He thought that they should have been paid less, because the populations they served were smaller and because their qualifications had not undergone the same scrutiny. Furthermore, grumbled Gregory, Clutsam and Eneas were only supposed to have been employed for three weeks, but their bills were for twice this term.[398] He referred their claims to the House of Assembly, where a select committee had been appointed to examine doctors' bills. The committee had already received the Nassau doctors' bills and had asked them to provide some supporting documentation. Chipman, in reply, had sent in a seven-feet-long scroll listing all of the medicines that had been supplied to the poor from his pharmacy. Gregory appended a note to the scroll, drawing the committee's attention to the fact that the doctors had charged the government the same rate as they charged private patients. Kirkwood's bill of £146 (equivalent to $21,472 today) was not held up for long. In June, the Council approved it for payment.[399]

The bills sent in to the governor came not only from doctors. The Board of Health needed another £58.7s (equivalent to $8,500 today) to cover miscellaneous epidemic-related expenses. Bills also came in from Harbour Island (see Appendix 4) including a claim from gravediggers Peter Saunders and Jacob Tynes, whose invoice was immediately rejected on the basis that it conflicted with some prior agreement. The Council expanded its clampdown. Mr Mardenbough, the Harbour Island receiver, was told to terminate the rental of Mrs Sarah Lowe's house in Dunmore Town that was being used as a cholera hospital.

The remaining outstanding bills were settled and the Council returned to the mundane business of running the colony, with no further mention of the epidemic. The newspapers did the same, padding their pages with stories vacuumed up from throughout the British Empire.

* * *

Governor Gregory's fear that he was reintroducing yellow fever to the colony when he returned from his vacation was tragically realised. The ill travellers had the yellow fever virus in their blood. Local *Aedes aegypti* mosquitos that bit them became infected and began to spread the disease. It took a while before anyone realised that a new epidemic was beginning. Captain Mostyn of the West India Regiment became an early victim. On Sunday, July 24, Governor Gregory attended his funeral. *The Nassau Guardian* editor wrote the following about the event.

> We cannot refrain from expressing our sorrow at the sudden death of Captain Mostyn, of H. M. 3rd West India regiment, whose arrival in this island we so recently announced. Captain Mostyn was taken ill of fever on Wednesday last, and died on the night of Saturday. He was buried with military honors on Sunday afternoon. His Excellency the Governor, accompanied by his Aides-de-camp, several members of Council, and other gentlemen, besides all the officers of the Garrison, attended at the interment of the highly-esteemed officer, so prematurely and unfortunately hurried to his grave amid all the regrets of all who knew him.[400]

On the evening of the funeral, Gregory developed a splitting headache and then a fever. Six days later, he died at Government House. *The Nassau Guardian* editor wrote the notice.

> It is our painful duty to record this evening the melancholy intelligence of the death of our highly respected Governor. His Excellency was attacked with fever on the night of Monday last and was considered by his medical attendant, the Hon. Dr. Kirkwood, who was called in on Tuesday, to be dangerously ill. The day after, Wednesday, the fever subsided and the most sanguine hopes were entertained of His Excellency's recovery. On Thursday, however, a change for the worse took place and another physician, the Hon. Dr. Chipman, was called in for the purpose of consultation. The most unremitting attention was bestowed by [them] that medical skill could devise for the recovery of the Governor, all of which proved unfortunately unavailing. His Excellency gradually declined until yesterday afternoon, when he breathed his last.

Gregory's post-mortem examination confirmed that he had been healthy up to the point of his sudden fatal illness.[401] It was an illness that would claim a succession of newcomers in a slow-burning epidemic that would drag on for a decade. It had not yet reached an alarming level when Sir Alexander Bannerman, the new governor, gave his first speech to House of Assembly. His remarks focused on the recent cholera epidemic. He shared his awareness of how miasmas were formed and he placed the risk of a recurrent epidemic squarely at the feet of the poor of Grants Town.

> I was then rejoiced to learn that the Colony had been particularly healthy since 1852, having recovered from the

> ravages of that malady, which, I understand, had proved so fatal to Grant Town, and the adjacent village at that period, nor could be otherwise, in localities where sewerage by ordinary means seems impracticable, and the lanes leading to the cottages, and dwellings, more apt to be choked with garbage preventing a free circulation of air, and becoming receptacles for all sorts of animal and vegetable matter, subject to the influence of a scorching sun, the exhalations from which are so prejudicial to health.
>
> I embrace this public opportunity of alluding to the subject, because although we cannot be too grateful to Divine Providence for the blessings we now enjoy, we know not how soon we may be re-visited by the cholera; and it is our imperative duty, by all the means in our power to endeavor to mitigate the increased evils which invariably follow in the train of that fatal epidemic, if we neglect those sanitary precautions which are always resorted to, but often when it is too late. Bannerman at the opening of Parliament. February 7, 1855.[402]

After this address, the government hardly mentioned the epidemic. It came up in 1857, in the government's call for tenders to build a wall around the cholera burial ground at Fortune Island.[403] This remote slip of land, now called Long Cay and located a mile south of Crooked Island, was where that island's victims of the epidemic found their final resting place.

Smallpox had by then overtaken cholera as the disease whose importation was most feared. Unlike the question mark that hung over the transmission of cholera and yellow fever, smallpox was unquestionably a contagious disease. In 1857, the Quarantine Station on Athol Island was under construction as an essential part of the government's strategy to keep the disease out.[404] And the memory of the cholera epidemic began to fade.

* * *

The colony would have done well to register the lessons offered up by the epidemic, but secondary events and the loss of key personnel interfered. The yellow fever epidemic, the loss of the *William and Mary* and the death of the governor himself afforded ample distraction.

Gregory's sudden departure had no apparent effect on the conduct of the colony's business, but his perspective in the aftermath would have been welcome had he been able to share it. Gavin's official report to the Colonial Office proved a crucial resource. Considering the cloud that covered his departure, the local administration would not have been inclined to correspond on his report, if it was even read. Dr Black, the port health officer, disappeared after the epidemic and the only other first-hand descriptions of events written in the immediate aftermath came from just two individuals.

On March 7, 1853, Dr Chipman wrote a letter to the editor of the *Association Medical Journal*. In it, he was cautiously optimistic that cholera was gone for good, as he mulled over its cause. He was clearly influenced by the opinion of the medical inspector, who had opined that cholera had been present in the colony in its so-called 'mild form' for at least a year before the big outbreak. Chipman, loath to contradict the inspector, gingerly distanced himself from those who were pointing accusatory fingers at the arrival of the *Reform*.

> I am happy to say that it has now entirely left our shores although probably, as in other instances, it may again revisit us. The mode of its introduction, whether by importation or otherwise, is involved in much obscurity. The general belief among the non-professional is, that it was introduced here by the schooner *Reform*, a vessel belonging to this port, and which had conveyed a cargo of pineapples to New York in August last. She lost a man from cholera while in the port of New York, but the disease did not extend to any of her crew, and she reached this island in September and was undergoing some cleansing in the vicinity of the spot where the disease first manifested itself. I cannot myself think that she had anything whatever to do with its introduction.[405]

Chipman's exculpation of the captain lacked conviction. He recounted the facts: that no cholera had been diagnosed in the colony before the return of the *Reform*; that the ship had lost a man to the disease during its visit to New York; that the first known victim in the colony had been Ann Hall, who had been well until September 17, when she suddenly died of cholera after having visited Captain Evans. In his mind, it was clear where the evidence was pointing.[406]

Chipman barely alluded to the blow that he had suffered when he lost his wife at the height of the epidemic. All that he had to say about his struggle was, 'How we got through the work, God only knows, but we were wonderfully preserved during a most arduous duty which occupied us night and day.'

He remarried, to Cecile (née Munnings), with whom he had several more children.[407] His career included pioneering the use of anaesthesia in The Bahamas, as indicated by his public demonstration of the use of nitrous oxide gas in 1851.[408] In 1864, his son, John F. H. Chipman, joined him in medical practice from Apothecaries Hall on Frederick Street, which was only a short walk from his home.[409] Chipman never wrote about the cholera epidemic again. Twenty years after the event, on June 13, 1873, weakened by a 'lingering and painful illness', he scratched out a barely legible signature at the bottom of the will that he dictated to his attorney, George C. Anderson, then Speaker of the House of Assembly. He died four weeks later, on July 17, 1873, at the age of sixty-nine.[410] His legacy includes an expansive family of high achievers. His grandson, Howard Nelson Chipman (1888–1951), who founded Chippingham, a residential community west of the City of Nassau, was buried next to him in the Western Cemetery. His great grandsons, Howard Nelson Chipman II and John 'Chippie' Chipman MBE (1928–2019), added local fame to the family name,[411] and his great-great grandson, Howard Nelson 'Chips' Chipman III, is a board-certified emergency medicine specialist, notable jet pilot and friend of the author.

Farre's experience of the epidemic was published in the *Medical Times and Gazette* the same month that Chipman's letter appeared in the *Association Medical Journal*. He wrote nothing more after this one report – and neither, it seems, did anyone else. A search for secondary sources on the governors, officials and eminent citizens of the day proved to be an exercise in futility. Investigators like myself have to face the fact that past historians downplayed the role of individuals as agents of change.[412] Only in the twenty-first century did the practice of documenting one's personal involvement in national events become accepted and encouraged.

Frederick Duncome, the one-time secretary to the short-lived Bahama Medical Board, resumed his busy civic and private-practice responsibilities. He remained a Member of Parliament for nearly twenty years. His epidemic experience no doubt informed his duties as a member of the Board of Public Works and the Board of Education. When he died on March 22, 1882 at the age of sixty-six, flags on all government buildings and forts were lowered to half-mast because he was, at the time, a sitting member of the Legislative Council.[413] *The Nassau Guardian* wrote the following.

> The passing away of such a distinguished gentleman, who being so prominently before the public for the past 40 years, deserves more than an ordinary notice. Shortly after his return from Edinburgh, where he had gained several high honors for his success in the examinations of medicine and surgery, Dr. Duncombe became a public man. Devoted to his profession, in all branches of which he was eminently skillful, he soon acquired a large practice. In 1854, he officiated as Health Officer, and in 1869 held that appointment in conjunction with the combined offices of Physician to the Prison and Police.

His obituary revealed significant changes that had been made to the health administration in the wake of the cholera epidemic. Notably, the post of medical inspector had been incorporated into its regular structure and its appointee was no longer a doctor sent from England. The obituary continued as follows.

> [H]e discharged the duties of Medical Inspector of the Colony, and as such as *ex-officio* Chairman of the Board of Health. He succeeded the Hon. Dr. Chipman, in 1873, as Medical Attendant at the Asylum, which post he held until 1880, when, in order to bring into effect arrangements contemplated for the better government of that institution, he was appointed resident surgeon superintendent of the Asylum; thus combining the medical department with that of General Superintendent of the entire establishment. Only two days before he died he resigned this office.

The obituary extolled the doctor's intellect and piety and applauded his contribution to the Christ Church Sunday School and Church Hall.

> Few men are as gifted with the versatile talents enjoyed by Dr. Duncombe. Having a remarkably retentive memory, he thoroughly mastered every subject which he took up. The lectures on astronomy, chemistry, and other kindred subjects, which he delivered before the Bahama Institute, manifest careful study, great research, and a profound depth of thought. With a wonderful command of language –

although at times quaint and original – he had the happy faculty of impressing his hearers by his earnestness. Above all, Dr. Duncombe was a truly pious Christian man. Like Timothy, he had served God from his youth, and his knowledge of the Scriptures was most extensive. For upwards of thirty years he superintended the Christ Church Sunday School, at the same time holding the office of Church-warden in the Vestry of that Parish, the Treasurer-ship first of the Bahama Church Society and subsequently of the Diocesan Council also of the colonial and Continental Church Society; he was a most valuable member of the church Synod, of which body he was also Chairman of Committees. It was mainly through his instrumentality that the Church Hall was built in 1849, having subscribed most liberally himself, and thereby induced others to follow his laudable example. He also gave a handsome donation towards the Endowment Fund of Christ Church, shortly after the passing of the prospective Disendowment Act, and up to the time of his last illness liberally supported, both by his means and influence all Diocesan and Parochial works. Nor did he confine his usefulness to his own Communion. He was for many years a hearty worker, as a member of the Committee of the Bahamas' Auxiliary of the British and Foreign Bible Society, on whose platform he as delivered many a telling speech. Dr. Duncombe was enrolled a member of the St. Andrews's Society in 1852, and in 1873 was elected President. This office he held continuously until the day of his death.[414]

Hector Gavin, the most likely of the frontliners to have written a memoir on The Bahamas epidemic, never had the opportunity to do so. Undoubtedly, it would have included an account of his experience in The Bahamas, but after leaving the colony he travelled to Trinidad and then to Grenada for a month or two, before returning to England. In September 1853, he was in Newcastle, where he was helping to manage a cholera outbreak. 'Purely out of courtesy', he summoned the local doctors to a meeting where he outlined his plan to tackle the epidemic. His approach went over badly, to say the least, and the meeting degenerated into insults and name-calling.

The clash with his colleagues triggered a formal enquiry but Gavin did not tarry for the outcome. As the epidemic raced to its ultimate toll of over 1,500 lives, he helped with displaced persons and burials, organised tents and monitored waste removal. And then he left. In November, he was in Dundee, promoting house-to-house visitation for cholera control as the city grappled with its outbreak. While there, he remarked on the uncleanliness of its residents. Their hygiene, he said, 'was worse than that of newly arrived Africans. Worse even than the nastiest of them all, the Portuguese.' The press picked up Gavin's offensive remark and, once again, the tactless busybody attracted the ire of the authorities.[415]

Gavin quit Dundee and in December was in his hometown of Edinburgh, visiting his father. By the time returned to London, Britain was at war in Crimea. It had begun in October 1853, when Britain attacked Russia, ostensibly over its incursions into the Balkans. Florence Nightingale, a social activist and amateur statistician who became famous for her role in professionalising nursing, travelled to the war zone on November 4, 1854. She arrived with a group of twenty nurses and they were headquartered at the Scutari Barrack Hospital. Even though they were badly needed, the doctors at first refused to allow them to help with any of the hospital's 1,500 patients.[416] The place was emblematic of all of the area's military hospitals, which were overcrowded and filthy death traps. Soldiers admitted with non-life-threatening injuries were dying in hospital from cholera, dysentery and scurvy. The wards were suffocating great rooms with low ceilings and few, tiny windows, and they were overrun with rats. The inadequate number of male military caregivers lacked sufficient clothing and eating utensils to distribute, which forced the nearly naked solders to eat from dirty bowls with grimy fingers. Nightingale recorded everything she saw and shared it in a stream of letters to influential friends back in England. The statistics that she kept proved beyond any shadow of doubt that military hospitals were far deadlier than any battlefield. Her letter-writing campaign caused the creation of a sanitary commission, charged with putting an end to the outrage of deadly military hospitals.

Hector Gavin volunteered to join the commission, which was led by John Sutherland, a highly respected physician, and included Robert Rawlinson, an eminent civil engineer. The trio arrived at Scutari, Crimea on March 6, 1855 and found a cholera epidemic raging in the Barrack Hospital. The hospital's sewer drains were blocked and the porous walls were saturated with the sewage that soaked the foundation. The commissioners whitewashed the walls, removed garbage and buried the bloated dead dogs putrefying about the yard. Rawlinson unblocked the sewer, put in filters, covered the storage tanks and created windows. The effect was dramatic and Nightingale later hailed their work as having saved the army.[417]

In April, the commissioners visited Balaclava, where Hector Gavin's younger brother, William, was stationed as veterinarian to a cavalry regiment. On April 20, Hector and a Dr Linton had dinner with William in his hut. Hector was inexperienced with firearms and nervous about the army standard-issue Deane and Adams five-shot revolver that he had been given. He asked William to keep the gun for him overnight. At around 10:30 p.m., they walked to the doorway and were at the threshold when Hector handed the weapon to his brother. Sutherland, the head commissioner, had the grim duty of writing to their father about what happened next.[418]

> Dr. Gavin was heard to say to his brother, 'William, you had better take my revolver with you tonight, and bring down the other in the morning'. He then went and took the revolver from the case. It was capped and loaded. He put his hand on William's shoulder and passed the pistol into William's hand, when it exploded so instantaneously that the servant stated it was impossible to tell in whose hand it had gone off. The shot passed though the left side of the abdomen and came out behind. The doctor said that he felt he was mortally wounded. Two military surgeons were on the spot in a quarter of an hour, and I saw him about the same time. There could be no doubt he had sustained a mortal injury. He lingered on till half-past seven o'clock this morning and died.[419]

William was devastated with grief from the accident, but not for long. Just eighteen days later, he died in Crimea of cholera. Gavin Milroy, the medical inspector who had gone to Jamaica, replaced Hector in Crimea.

Milroy was known as a writer, but he left no memoir on his time in the West Indies. Neither did Charles Nesbitt, the top civil servant in The Bahamas. He would have been an ideal author for a report on the once-in-a-century event, but after his retirement in 1867, he lived out his years in New Providence. He died at the age of seventy-seven at his home on Bay Street on December 15, 1876, and was buried in St Mary's Churchyard.

❧ ❧ ❧

After The Bahamas cholera epidemic, all mention of it dropped from the news until fourteen years later, when, in September of 1866, New Providence was devastated by a hurricane. The storm killed 387 people and destroyed over 1,000 buildings, including the Quarantine Station. The *Reform*, which had brought cholera to the colony, was one of the 300 vessels reported damaged.[420] *The Nassau Guardian* alluded to the epidemic in its reporting on the hurricane.

> A number of human bones are to be seen on the sands, from Roslyn westwardly to an indefinite extent. *The Cholera Burial ground is intact*, therefore either some long-forgotten burial-place must have been encroached upon by the waves, or perhaps they themselves have given up what was consigned to the deep.[421]

The newspaper recalled the cholera epidemic of just fourteen years earlier as if it was ancient history. The ghostly memory was reburied with bones and forgotten again for another twenty years. In 1884, when cholera once again erupted in Europe, the memory of The Bahamas epidemic was recalled by Governor Blake. He feared the colony might not be spared, as it had been with the epidemic that hit America in 1860s. To arm residents with knowledge on disease prevention, he enlisted the local medical fraternity to deliver a series of public lectures. The talks were published in a booklet titled 'How to Avoid Fever, Consumption or Cholera: Papers on Sanitation', with Kirkwood as the first speaker.[422] He was followed by three Bahamian medical graduates of the University of Pennsylvania. George Kemp (1832–1901), whose practice was also located on Frederick Street, spoke on 'Overcrowding and Ventilation'. J. Benson Albury (1842–1910), who was just a boy when the colony was battling cholera, lectured on the 'Impurity of Water and Its Remedies'. William Maclure (1839–1900), who was the son of the Reverend Maclure, spoke on the 'Evils of Weeds and Bush'. A fifth speaker, Dr William Robinson, gave a lecture titled 'The Value of Earth as a Deodorizer and of Lime as a Disinfectant'.

Kirkwood was seventy years old at the time and the only remaining physician who had fought on the front line during the cholera epidemic. He had long retired from government service and given up his administrative duties, which at one point saw him simultaneously serving as chairman of six public boards. He had enjoyed a sojourn of seven years in Italy, indulging his love of art. Kirkwood was himself reportedly a decent artist, and the walls of his house were lined with copies that he had made of famous paintings. Although retired, Kirkwood was still a force. Upon his return from Italy in 1879, Governor Robinson reappointed him to the Legislative Council, and he was president of the St Andrew's Society. Kirkwood's lecture, 'General Principles of Sanitation', began as follows.

> The subject of Sanitation is very large, and the time allotted to each speaker is very short, so I must necessarily confine myself to the most prominent causes of disease immediately surrounding us, in the air we breathe, in the water we drink – elements so essential to health and life, and when impure so detrimental to both. It may be laid down as an axiom that polluted air and water are the causes of a great proportion of the disease of humanity.

Kirkwood made an astounding revelation in his talk. All the way back in 1853, he had deduced that cholera was caused by drinking water and not by an airborne poison.

> The fatal consequences resulting from the use of impure water was strikingly manifested during the same [cholera] epidemic. Soon after its appearance in the island, the men of the Garrison resident in Barracks with their families, were ordered to be strictly confined therein, though in good health at the time. In a few days, however, a violent outbreak of cholera took place, which disease continued to rage until it was deemed advisable to permit the free egress of the surviving inmates.

> Why so violent an outbreak should have taken place in a building so admirably situated for heath, so spacious, so well ventilated, and so thoroughly clean, and grounds perfectly free from any injurious matters? I pondered over this, to me, apparent puzzle for a long time – two or three months in fact; when it occurred to me to enquire into the character of the water used by the inhabitants of the Barracks during the period of their confinement. I found that they had always used for drinking and culinary purposes the water from a well in the adjoining Ordnance yard, of good quality, of which they were deprived, and restricted to the use of the water in the wells in the Barrack yard, which was impure and brackish to a degree quite sufficient to account for the evils resulting from its use. The puzzle was solved, and left me without a doubt that in all probability no cholera would have attacked the people in Barracks if the unfortunate mistake of confining them to the use of bad water had not been made.[423]

He continued.

> I am strengthened and confirmed in this opinion by the fact that cholera, as far as the Garrison was concerned, confined itself exclusively to the inmates of the Barracks, and the rest of the Garrison were in no instance affected by it. The Officers' Quarters, you all know, are not distant more than a very few yards from the Barracks, but no officer suffered, although in daily contact with cholera patients in their visitations to the Hospital. None of their servants, not a

> nurse or orderly resident in the Hospital suffered in the slightest degree from the fell destroyer.[424]

Kirkwood's insight was decades ahead of this becoming general knowledge. In the 1990s, Charles Rosenberg observed from his studies of epidemics how in medicine, accepted wisdom changed slowly, 'not necessarily in the minds of a few great men, but in the substrate of assumption ... which constitutes the intellectual texture of an age'.[425] Kirkwood's mind was one of the great ones, but he had no intention of rocking the boat or exposing himself to ridicule, which was a real risk. His perception came at a time when the notion that cholera was a waterborne disease was a fringe idea. Kirkwood realised this even before John Snow's dramatic demonstration with the Broad Street pump handle in Soho.[426] The miasma theory only collapsed in 1882, after Robert Koch isolated the cholera bacillus from victims in Egypt. Kirkwood may have privately shared what he had perceived, but he kept his knowledge a secret from the public for thirty-two years.

The elderly doctor extolled the virtues of fresh air, and the advice he gave in 1884 remains applicable today for the prevention of airborne infections. He wrote the following.

> One of the most common and most easily preventable causes of disease in our island is vitiated air, arising from want of ventilation in sleeping apartments, in which a number of people shut themselves up with every door, window and cranny closed, exhaling poisonous carbonic acid gas, and re-breathing it over and over again, poisoning their blood an

> sapping their health – laying the foundations of disease ten, ay a thousand times more fatal than cholera – I mean pulmonary consumption. This self-poisoning is persevered in because the delusion exists that night air is injurious, a widespread fallacy not confined to the Bahamas. Night air is not injurious, and in fact it contains more oxygen and less noxious foreign matters in large cities than day air.
>
> One of the most potent remedial agents in the treatment of disease is constant and thorough ventilation. Think of this when you shut the doors and windows of a sick room, crowd into it a number of visitors, and, with the best and kindest intentions in the world, do your best to kill the patient or at least impede his or her recovery.[427]

He let it be known that he had little confidence in quarantine.

> I cannot too strongly urge upon you how necessary and beneficial are the measures just pointed out, cholera, or no cholera. A visitation from that dreadful enemy is a mere possibility; but the presence of other diseases, incidental to our climate and the poisonous causes I have enumerated is a certainty. Trust in Sanitation and not in Quarantine; the first has always proved successful in limiting or preventing the spread of epidemic diseases, the last has always failed most signally.

Kirkwood died childless four years later, on December 9, 1888, of heart disease. His demise came just three months after losing

Abby, his wife of fifty-two years.[428] He outlived his buddies, Maclure (died 1863) and Moseley (died 1885), whose sons became the executors of his estate. *The Nassau Guardian* lauded the physician in its obituary.[429]

> When in practice, he was most generous to the poor, and especially to those who through misfortune were in reduced circumstances. During the epidemic of cholera in 1852, he was instant in season and out of season in administering relief to all who sought his aid, whether he was likely to receive compensation for his services or not.

Kirkwood left sums to St Andrew's Presbyterian Church, to his godson and to friends, including his housemaid and to this 'old and faithful cook'. However, the bulk of his estate was sold to create a trust for women in Nassau 'of good character and respectability' who had fallen on hard times.[430] As trustees, he designated the Reverend Robert Dunlop of St Andrew's Kirk (and his successors), the Reverend Robert Swan, rector of Christ Church (and his successors) and Mr John Sargent Darling, a Nassau merchant.

In 1889, Edward George, the son of Deacon John S. George, purchased Cascadilla, which was conveniently less than half a block from John S. George Hardware, a store on Bay Street that he owned and managed.[431] Later, it became the town home of Sir Harold Christie and Lady Christie, whose main residence was in Lyford Cay. They preserved the set-up of Kirkwood's clinic, but after it was sold again it was allowed to decay and collapse.[432]

Kirkwood's estate lives on, however, with a residuum that provides a modest income to the needy to this day.[433]

I believe that the colony's administrators forgot the traumatic cholera epidemic on purpose, and that they did so by silence and negation.[434] By this means, the government was able to avoid criticism for its lack of planning, for breaking its own rules, for housing emigrant refugees in the deadly barracks, for flip-flopping on burial instructions and for other errors. Medical Inspector Gavin had been called by his superiors in London to explain how he had failed to quarantine the yellow-fever-ridden *Esk*. In this, the local doctors and the governor were complicit. Now, with yellow fever spreading in the colony, the administration was likely keen not to add this new epidemic to the mistakes for which it might have to account. In addition, the tenor of the Executive Council discussions surrounding the sums paid for healthcare during the epidemic made it clear that the administration had no intention of sustaining, much less expanding, the services it had introduced on an emergency basis. The colony had neither the money nor the desire to improve the lot of former slaves. By avoiding a discussion of the epidemic, it allowed the improvements and services that Gavin had urged to evaporate. The remarkable William Kirkwood avoided rocking the boat. He kept mum on the insights that he had gained regarding the transmission of cholera by contaminated water from the outbreak in the garrison. The rich and powerful doctor never used his influence to steer health policy. Consequently, the Board of Health never faced any opposition to its fixation on the miasma theory, which so well leant itself to the leadership's propensity to blame its primary victims.

It seems that the government found two excuses that sustained its intent to downplay and forget the disaster. Firstly, the epidemic in The Bahamas was not as bad as that suffered by its neighbours. The one in Jamaica dragged on for two years and killed an estimated 40,000 persons. The mortality of the epidemic in Barbados, which ran from May through November 1854, was comparable with Jamaica's, and it caused a secondary crisis through the multitude of orphans that resulted.[435] Even at that level of mass extermination, *The Barbadian* managed to parse a positive angle.

> [F]or whilst 18,009 of our population has been taken off, no want of labour has as yet been experienced, and many whose lives were before spent in utter inactivity, have turned to work, and promise in the end to become valuable labourers. The attendance, too, at church as very perceptibly increased, and it is hoped that, as this feeling increases, it will bring forth such fruits as will render this a more happy community than it has hitherto been, owning to the unsettled state of our labourers' minds, and their constant bickerings and contentions with one another, as well as with those above them.[436]

Trinidad and St Lucia faced similarly devastating epidemics, as did St Kitts, where an estimated 3,000 died of its population of 24,000.[437] The Bahamas epidemic was tame by comparison. The ruling elite may have believed that The Bahamas had a better health system, or less poisonous air.

Secondly, a difference in how the disease spread in New Providence at the outset allowed the local elite to invoke a racist rationalisation that they were relatively protected. Cholera's first victims in The Bahamas were White residents, and twenty-four of them died (see Appendix 2), but it killed some 1,200 people in total. The leadership embraced the dogma that Black people were weaker, dirtier, immoral and more easily panicked – all attributes that attracted the disease to them and worsened the outcome. These racist views prevailed throughout the British Empire, but the belief was especially detrimental to Bahamians because the leadership dismissed the squalor of the poor as being devoid of any personal threat. By contrast, the epidemics in Jamaica and Barbados began in their Black communities. Jamaican and Bajan authorities had to see that the conditions in their dark-skinned brethren posed a threat to the health of everyone. The differing perspectives led to different post-epidemic outcomes. Jamaica enacted many of the health improvements that Inspector Milroy had recommended, and it began soon after the epidemic. Barbados formed the Bridgetown Waterworks Company within the decade[438] and, by 1861, Bridgetown had piped clean water.[439]

Cholera struck Hamilton, Ontario and Barbados in the same year. Hamilton, which lost 5 per cent of its residents to the epidemic, also immediately began planning a waterworks. Both cities celebrated the achievement of clean water and pressurised fire hydrants, with the construction of decorative city-centre water fountains. In 1860, the Gore Park Fountain in Hamilton was dedicated and, in 1865, Barbados followed with the Dolphin Fountain in Bridgetown. Neither city explicitly mentioned the cholera epidemic that triggered the creation of the monuments. However, in their trumpeting of modernity and cleanliness, they stood as positive outcomes of a destructive epidemic.[440]

The Bahamas did nothing about its health services in the wake of the epidemic, and a full seventy years passed before the colony moved to provide a clean water supply for New Providence. When it finally did so, the decision had nothing to do with cholera. The yellow fever epidemic that followed cholera dragged on until the end of the 1800s. At the turn of the twentieth century, typhoid fever replaced it as the number-one public health hazard.

Unlike the confusion that surrounded the origin of the cholera epidemic, in 1900, the year the House of Assembly appointed a select committee to discuss building a clean water supply system for Nassau, there was no question about the origin of typhoid. The House was no more ready to spend money on health then than it had been during the cholera epidemic. The committee never reported and allowed the matter to die. In 1912, the complaints of American visitors revived the call for clean water. In July 1913, Dr McHattie, the chief medical officer, noted a surge in typhoid cases and urged action. This caused Governor Haddon-Smith to ask the secretary of state to send an expert engineer to design and price a system for Nassau. The special danger to visitors was used as a carrot.

> [A] real danger lies in the fact that a considerable number of visitors come to Nassau every year, attracted by its cleanness magnificent climate: these visitors are accustomed to a pure

> water supply, and are therefore much more liable to contract disease than the inhabitants themselves …
>
> There have been out-breaks of illness in various health resorts and the effect of such outbreaks is too well known to require any comment.[441]

The risk of a devastating fire was also very much on the governor's mind. Most of the city's buildings were made of wood and some were very large. A piped water supply would have been a major asset to fire safety. To buttress his case for the expenditure, which he knew the House of Assembly would resist, he ordered water samples from around Nassau to be sent to England for analysis.[442] In January 1914, the laboratory reported that all of the well water samples tested were unfit for human consumption. That May, H. Howard Humphreys, the water engineer sent out from London, submitted his report, 'Proposed Waterworks for the City of Nassau'. It called for water to be sourced at the Blue Hills and pumped to a tower near the city. He was conscious of the aesthetics of the plan, writing the following.

> In order to show that a water tower need not of necessity be objectionable in appearance, the design for a structure which can be built almost entirely of local stone has been prepared. The character of this tower is in keeping with the masonry of Fort Fincastle. Humphreys, May 18th, 1914.

Humphreys identified the major arguments opposing expenditure on a waterworks. Lawmakers claimed that there had never been a serious outbreak of waterborne disease in the colony, revealing their complete ignorance of the 1852 cholera epidemic. They argued that there had never been a disastrous fire, and they said that most people drank the water with no apparent ill-effects, regardless of whatever the scientists in England thought of the colony's water samples.[443] They shelved Humphreys' proposal and allowed typhoid and other waterborne diseases to continue unchecked.

Almost a decade passed before the issue came up again. McHattie's successor, Alexander Pearce, blasted the Board of Health over the conditions that had been allowed to persist. He was exasperated by the fact that just one sanitary inspector was employed for the whole of New Providence. A tour of 300 homes, from Church Street, not far from where the cholera outbreak had begun, westward through the city to Victoria Avenue, left him fuming.

> My experiences during the past week have surpassed anything I imaged possible to exist and twice owing to the odours and filth I encountered, I became ill and had to retire from work for the afternoon. I finished my tour of inspection with an infected throat, which is only now getting better.
>
> Chaos and filth predominated in most of the yards. Barrels unprotected and full of mosquito larvae, water tanks and wells not properly covered, privies open and not fly screened. In the majority of cases these were full of water, broken down and in dangerous proximity to wells and dwelling houses.

> You will also notice on perusing the detailed report that overcrowding exists among the poorer classes in several special areas. The majority of these people keep pigs, goats and sheep. The pigs are usually kept in pens that are not properly decked and cleaned. The resulting quagmire surpasses description, with its accompanying odour and flies. A. Pearce, July 1923.[444]

Even this condemnation failed to move the executive. The tipping point was only reached in 1927, when yet another outbreak of typhoid fever killed a tourist in New Providence. The government commissioned Sir Wilfred Beveridge, a London School of Tropical Medicine expert, to give advice. Beveridge chided the authorities, who were clearly more interested in protecting the fledgling tourist economy than in health. He wrote the following.

> There appears to be a desire on the part of the Board of Health to avoid undue publicity in connection with the present prevalence of typhoid. This, I think, is a wrong attitude to take. The fact that any serious infectious disease is present should be made known to the people, and posters and pamphlets should be issued pointing out the seriousness of the disease, the manner in which the disease is contracted, and the measures to be taken by the community to avoid infection and to limit the spread of the disease. It is far better to take the people into one's confidence and invite their aid than to try to disguise the presence of an infectious disease, which, in a campaign of prevention, leads us nowhere.[445]

Beveridge was spot-on. The Board of Health in 1852 had done a much better job of it than this one. It had freely shared statistics and repeatedly published the treatments recommended by the experts. Beveridge went on to warn the government that another explosive outbreak of typhoid could happen at any moment, and this, at last, got the leadership to move with speed. By the end of 1928, it had built the system that Humphreys had designed: an 80,000-gallon water tank atop a 126-feet-tall tower made of reinforced concrete and erected on the highest point on New Providence. The tower was painted white and its crown-like head was topped by a navigation beacon, which blinked like a jewel as it revolved.

The new water system was too little and too late for Frances Stoddard, the new wife of a prominent New Haven banker. She died in Nassau of typhoid contracted while on vacation, mere months after the tower was commissioned.[446] Even after her death, the system expanded so slowly that a decade later it still only served a small section of the community – mainly the well-off residents of Nassau.[447] It was 1963 before the majority of New Providence households had abandoned the use of backyard wells for public standpipes. Unsurprisingly, waterborne diseases retreated just as slowly. In 1965, three deaths from amoeba infestation were reported and, in 1973, nine children died of dysentery.[448] Even in the 1980s, when the author was an intern at the Princess Margaret Hospital, amoeba parasitic infestation was still common.[449] Those diseases are gone now and, though unappreciated by the general public, those who administer the city's waterworks have celebrated what was achieved. In 1993, The

Bahamas Water and Sewerage Corporation declared the Water Tower a national water landmark.[450]

The magnificent landmark is ignored and the availability of clean drinking water that it triumphantly broadcasts is taken for granted in The Bahamas. Few are aware of the warning contained in the 2006 US Army Corps of Engineers study that called attention to the peril faced by the nation's water supply from climate change and sea-level rise. The Corps' report pointed out that many of the fragile freshwater lenses on New Providence were already impaired. Numerous lenses had been contaminated by sewerage, harmed by fuel leaks and spoiled by salt-water intrusion and collective over-pumping, from an estimated (at the time) 30,000 private wells.[451] The report supported the Water and Sewerage Corporation's call for water to be regarded as a strategic national resource, so that the people of this nation do not join the 2.4 billion people around the world who, according to the World Health Organization, do not have ready access to clean water.

Cholera still sickens 3 million persons and kills some 95,000 every year. Thousands have died in recent epidemics in Yemen, the Democratic Republic of the Congo, Somalia and South Sudan, in addition to the outbreak in neighbouring Haiti.

The ongoing epidemic in Haiti has created a reservoir of cholera in the region.[452] Normal trade has always been sufficient to disperse the disease. The turmoil in Haiti has heightened the danger by increasing the numbers of desperate migrants. Sooner or later, another will arrive in The Bahamas carrying cholera. Even if this person is intercepted and isolated, we know that this is no guarantee of protection. Safeguarding the nation's water supply is the only dependable strategy to prevent an outbreak.

❦ ❦ ❦

The Bahamas is not unique in its forgetting of the cholera epidemic. At Batt's Rock, Barbados sits perhaps the only memorial expressly dedicated to cholera victims in the Caribbean. Throughout the world there are scores more. Many mark mass graves – or cholera pits, as they were called – like the one in Ayrshire, Scotland. Most of them are over a century old, but a handful are new, like the 2017 Cholera Memorial at St Mary's, downtown Toronto. In The Bahamas, scraps of physical structures exist that that could serve as present-day reminders of the epidemic. Some of the 200-odd cuboid cholera gravestones placed by Sexton Roos in St Matthew's Graveyard are still there. Today they are painted white and arrayed as decoration along the graveyard's main walkway, with no indication of their original purpose. Remnants still exist of the graves at the Bethlehem yard, where a number of cholera victims were buried. Their stones fringe the margins of what is today a public playground at the corner of Meeting and Augusta Streets. The whereabouts of the cholera graves dug on the north side of Paradise Island is unknown and no one is sure where the cholera burial ground created to the west of the town, the one referred to in the wake of the 1866 hurricane, was located. Hope Town and Elbow Cay in the Abaco Islands have marked their cholera gravesites.

Nowhere in the West Indies is the disaster commemorated.

Epidemics, accidents and natural disasters, deemed acts of God, take more lives, but are easier for a community to reconcile. For instance, the fire and sinking of the *Yarmouth Castle* cruise ship in 1965, which took more than eighty souls to the bottom of the ocean near the Berry Islands, is scarcely remembered.[453] Every year thousands of tourists sail to and around the private playground built by a cruise line near the sinking, with no allusion to the mass grave below. Multiple other candidates for commemoration remain the province of the history buff and the scholar.

Deaths wrought deliberately, by contrast, are much harder to forgive and forget. More than forty years after Cuban MiG fighter jets attacked and sank the HMBS *Flamingo* and killed four Royal Bahamas Defence Force sailors, the nation remains shaken. In a solemn annual ceremony at the cenotaph in the city centre, the memory of the lost Defence Force sailors is honoured along with those soldiers killed in the two World Wars.

The cholera epidemics of the 1850s were the deadliest events in the region. In The Bahamas, the memory of the epidemic evaporated like the miasma from which it was believed to have sprung. Resurrecting it has shone a light on the poverty and the appalling living conditions endured by the recently emancipated residents. It has revealed how the uncaring government ignored and repressed them and how it failed at disaster management. An awareness of the lessons held forth by the experience is much more important than any possible future commemoration. It was such a hard lesson to allow to go completely to waste.

# Epilogue

In March of 2019, swarms of toads invaded areas of South Florida. Upscale homes in the city of Palm Beach Gardens were inundated with countless baby cane toads, also called bufos. Thousands of the dime-sized critters carpeted driveways, patios and lawns. It became impossible to step outside without smushing them underfoot. They clogged pool filters and created a booming business for pest removers, who netted, swept and vacuumed up the hoppers. Experts attributed the swarming of this invasive species of toad to changes in water oxygen levels, the unseasonably warm weather and the loss of fish. No one was foolish enough to suggest that the swarm could be a harbinger of an approaching epidemic.

On March 1, 2020, Governor Ron DeSantis announced that the first two Floridians had tested positive for coronavirus. Shortly thereafter, on March 15, it was announced that a sixty-one-year-old female resident of New Providence had become the first confirmed person with Covid-19 in The Bahamas. Thus began a regimen of quarantine, social distancing and sanitising everything we touched. Patients were prescribed the anti-malarial drug hydroxychloroquine and the anti-parasitic ivermectin, both of which were later proved to be of no benefit. Hospital experts advocated early ventilation for failing lungs, only to later discover that this procedure worsened outcomes. Freedom of movement, a right enjoyed under Article 25 of The Bahamas Constitution, was curtailed for the first time in the nation's history, in the interest of public health. The government gave the Ministry of Health money to hire additional contact-tracing personnel and to purchase testing supplies. Western Medical Plaza on Blake Road became a dedicated Covid-19 hospital.

In May, the month in which residents first experienced a series of nationwide lockdowns, the toads were spotted in New Providence. These were not the dime-sized baby bufos that had flooded the enclaves in Florida, but fully grown two-pound giants. A task force was deployed by the Department of Environmental Health to 'seek and destroy' the poison-secreting invaders.[454] The death toll from Covid-19 stood at fourteen when, in August, almost 400 toads had been caught.[455] A second wave of Covid-19 infections immediately began and it continued, with surges and ebbs, for three years. By 2023, some 38,000 persons had tested positive and 844 deaths had been directly attributed to the virus.

The stress of caring for so many seriously ill patients with this deadly infectious disease boiled over into healthcare worker unrest. Nurses complained about the delay in receiving hazard pay and emergency personnel staged a sickout. The local representative of the Inter-American Development Bank called the epidemic an 'unprecedented challenge' for most governments. It estimated that it cost the country $9.5 billion, but the economic pain was by no means evenly shared. The disaster was a windfall for private testing and treatment facilities. Doctors Hospital Ltd. alone enjoyed a quadrupling of its net income during the epidemic.

Similarities and parallels between the cholera epidemic and the current Covid-19 disaster continue to emerge. This really should come as no surprise. History does indeed repeat itself, and like the famous tragedies in theatre, which have been continually rewritten and retold, no matter how the details of the script are changed, those who know the original recognise the play.

# Appendix 1

*Recommended Treatments for Cholera*

*Source*: 'By Order of the Board. C.G. Wylly, Secretary. Bahamas Board of Health Notice'. *Bahama Herald* and *The Nassau Guardian*, September 25, 1852.

No. 1. Mix the following in a tablespoonful of gruel.

| | |
|---|---|
| • Camphor | 5 grains |
| • Opium | 1 grain |
| • Calomel | 10 grains |
| • Cayenne pepper | 2 grains |

No. 2. One hour after giving mixture number 1, commence mixture number 2.

| | |
|---|---|
| • Chalk mixture | 8 ounces |
| • Soda (carbonate) | 3 drachms |
| • Spirits of Camphor | 3 drachms |
| • Essences of Ginger | 3 drachms |
| • Laudanum | 3 drachms |

Mix. If quinine can be procured, add twenty grains. If the attack be severe, add 30 to 60 drops of tincture of catechu to each dose. Dose: A tablespoon every hour or two, until all uneasy symptoms be relieved. The person is to lie down perfectly still while using the medicine, persevering till relieved. At the same time, flannel, wet with turpentine, should be applied to the stomach, and if the limbs be cool, flannels wrung out of hot water, and sprinkled with mustard, are to be applied to the extremities. The indiscriminate use of brandy in such cases is not commendable.

In the course of a day or two, if the state of the bowels require it, a small dose of Castor-oil or Gregory's powder may be taken, resuming for a few days longer, the mixture in less frequent doses.

The daily use of some bitter tea, as Gentian, sweet-wood bark, or Colomba, with carbonate of soda, is recommended for convalescents, as well as for the healthy during the prevalence of Cholera.

IV. Every house should be furnished with blankets, flannel, mustard, turpentine, the means of procuring hot water with as little delay as possible, and also with a large tub or other vessel for administering a warm bath.

**Cholera Proper**

When the more formidable disease manifests itself, as may be recognized by either vomiting or purging, usually of rice-coloured evacuations, a burning heat at the stomach, with or without cramps in the bowels and limbs, and coldness of the surface:

1. A warm bed must be resorted to.

2. Warmth must be assiduously applied by means of heated flannels, hot water in bottles, or other more suitable vessels, bags of heated sand, ashes, bran, or salt, being placed at the feet, legs, sides and back.

3. Poultices of mustard should be applied previously to the abdomen for 20 or 30 minutes.

4. Steady and persevering frictions over the whole body and limbs, with spirits of turpentine and strong hartshorn.

5. The whole body and extremities may be enveloped in a sheet soaked in turpentine, a blanket thrown over, and frictions maintained outside.

**REMEDIES**

No. 3.

- Calomel 30 grains
- Opium 12 grains
- Camphor 12 grains
- Cayenne pepper 12 grains

Mix. Divide into 12 pills or powders, one of which should be given to adults every hour alternately, with a dose of the following:

No. 4.

- Chalk mixture 6 ounces
- Spirits of camphor 12 grains
- Laudanum 2 drachms
- Tincture of capsicum (red pepper) 1 drachm

| | |
|---|---|
| • Essence of peppermint | 1 ounce |
| • Carbonate of soda | 2 drachms |
| • Sulphate of quinine (if procurable) | 30 grains |

Mix. Dose – A tablespoonful every hour for adults. Children, one-half the quantity. A few drops of ether may be added to each dose, or where the mixture is not retained, may be given by itself in a little mint tea, and the mixture resumed. Injections of laudanum and arrowroot should be administered to allay the violent cramps.

It should be constantly borne in mind during the tendency to cholera epidemic, that the use of purgative medicine of a cold or drastic character, as salts, seidlitz powders, senna, & etc., is injurious. The best aperient medicines, when required, are castor-oil, Gregory's mixture, or the compound Rhubarb pill.

Families are recommended to provide themselves beforehand with everything requisite for the treatment of the disorder, as much valuable time may be lost, when the emergency arises, that might have been saved by a little foresight.

The following should be in readiness:

- A supply of blankets
- Spirits of turpentine, in bottles
- Bottles of mustard
- 1 ounce of carbonate of ammonia
- 2 ounces spirits of ammonia
- 2 ounces sulphuric ether
- 2 ounces laudanum

# Appendix 2

*Named Residents Who Died of Cholera**

1. Mrs Ann Hall. 'On Thursday September 16 after a few hours' illness, widow of the late Capt. John W. Hall, aged 53.' *Bahama Herald*, September 18, 1852.

2. Miss Rachael Armbrister in the Eastern District. 'Only daughter of John Armbrister Esq., of St. Salvador. Age 24, on Sunday September 19, 1852 after a few hours' illness.' *The Nassau Guardian*, September 25, 1852; *Bahama Herald*, September 22, 1852.

3. Mrs Sears, 'relict of the late David Sears Esq. of this town'. *The Nassau Guardian*, September 25, 1852.

4. Emily Susan Sears, 'daughter of the late David Sears', St. Andrews Presbyterian Church Sunday School teacher. *The Nassau Guardian*, September 25, 1852.

5. Mrs Sara Melissa Brice, aged fifty-two. *The Nassau Guardian*, September 25, 1852.

6. George Albert Brice, aged seventeen. *The Nassau Guardian*, September 25, 1852.

7. Esther Butler Claxton, 'age 52, on Wednesday 20th October of cholera, leaving a large circle of relatives and friends to lament her sudden removal'. *The Nassau Guardian*, October 27, 1852.

8. Mr William Mather, 'Foreman of the Ordnance yard, age 38, on October 26. A faithful public servant for sixteen years and highly respected in this community.' *The Nassau Guardian*, October 27, 1852.

9. 'On Saturday, 30th October, after a few hours' illness, of the prevailing epidemic, Glovina, youngest daughter of Mr. John Polhemus, aged 16 years'. 'Died'. *The Nassau Guardian*, November 3, 1852.

10. 'On Sunday morning 24th October in the 15th year of her age, Charlotte Mary Ann, eldest daughter of the late Hon. Geo. P. Wood; and, on the same day, her sister, in the 21st year of her age, Mary Jane, wife of George Allan, Esquire, Lieutenant in H.M. 1st WI Regiment and eldest daughter of the late John Lightbody Patterson, M.D., Surgeon Royal Navy'. 'Died'. *The Nassau Guardian*, November 3, 1852.

11. Amelia Catherine Maura, wife of the Spanish consul, November 17, 1852.

12. 'Yesterday, Ida Blanche, youngest child of Captain Craig, commanding H.M. 1st W.I. Regt., aged 7 ½ months'. 'Died'. *The Nassau Guardian*. November 20, 1852.

13. Mrs John Maura Jr., 'youthful partner of John Maura Junior Esquire, Acting Spanish Consul'. *The Nassau Guardian*, November 19, 1852.

14. Edmund Burnett, seaman on the *Esk*, November 22, 1852.

15. William Horne Gould, aged twenty-five years and eight months, 'late Revenue Officer at Rum Cay. Of amiable disposition, he has died in the prime of life'. 'Died'. *The Nassau Guardian*, December 4, 1852.

16. 'On Saturday evening last, after a few hours' illness, of cholera, Miss Isabella Carmichael, in the 60th years of her age.' 'Died'. *The Nassau Guardian*, December 11, 1852.

17. Joseph Bersch, aged twenty-one, on December 10. *Ovando* immigrant. *The Nassau Guardian*, December 15, 1852.

18. Margaretta Palm, aged fourteen, on December 14. *Ovando* immigrant. *The Nassau Guardian*, December 15, 1852.

19. Joseph Schneider, aged ten, on December 15. *Ovando* immigrant. *The Nassau Guardian*, December 15, 1852.

20. Miss Isabella Carmichael, aged sixty, 'of cholera after a few hours' illness on Saturday evening last'. *The Nassau Guardian*, December 11, 1852.

21. 'It is our painful duty to record, this evening, with deep regret – a regret which we are sure is shared in by the entire community – the sudden death of Miss Eliza Lees, the young and highly esteemed daughter of Chief Justice Lees.' 'Editorial'. *The Nassau Guardian*, December 22, 1852.

22. 'At Ragged Island on the 22nd December, Fanny Jane, only daughter of the Rev. W. H. and Maria E. Strombom, and on the 23rd Maria E., the beloved wife of the Rev. W. H. Strombom.** By this doubly afflicted dispensation, a fond husband and father is left to mourn his irreparable loss, together with a large circle of relatives and friends, to whom Mrs. Strombom was endeared by an amiablility of manner and character seldom equalled. In her death was displayed the full perfection of a ripe Christian, whose only hope was in her Redeemer, where her faith was superior to the strong ties that bound her to a fond Husband and her infant child, and rendered her exit to a better world a truly happy one.' 'Died'. *The Nassau Guardian*, January 19, 1853.

23. Rose Micklewhite, ordnance nurse. 'Editorial'. *The Nassau Guardian*, December 25, 1852.

24. Elizabeth Anna Turtle, aged twenty-seven, wife of Mr John J. Turtle and daughter of the late P. S. Lightbourne of

Nassau. Member of the Wesleyan Church from childhood. 'A few days' severe illness'. *The Nassau Guardian*, March 30, 1853.

*Only White residents were named in the newspapers. None of the 1,175-odd Black residents of the colony who died in the epidemic were identified in the press.

**Reverend William Henry Strombom (1816–1895), an Englishman, was rector at St Patrick's Anglican Church in Governor's Harbour, where residents had imposed an illegal quarantine. The embargo, which the government busted, as discussed in the text, may well have saved the reverend's life, as it prevented his family's return from Ragged Island. Strombom subsequently remarried, to Elizabeth Ann (née Duncombe), with whom he had twelve children. He was buried in St Matthew's Anglican Church Cemetery.

# Appendix 3

*Letters*

*From Dr Hector Gavin to his Excellency the Governor.*
*Minutes of the Executive Council,*
*Nassau, November 16, 1852*

Your Excellency, I have the honour to state for the information of your Excellency that having according to my instructions made myself acquainted with the measures which have been taken to prevent the spread of Epidemic Cholera among the people of this Island & Colony, I am of opinion that, with a view to the saving of human life, it is absolutely essential that the present constitution of the Board of Health should be changed, & that the medical men, who with one exception, are the same persons who transact the business of the Board, should be relieved from the onerous and improper functions now entailed on them, in relation to matters in —wise connected with their profession but which engross much of their time to the injury of the Public, who should during the present epidemic have, as far as practicable, their unrestricted services.

I have further to object to the constitution of the Board that in matters of finance they are called upon to certify their own accounts.

I have to state that although very valuable and important considerations were submitted by the Board of Health to the Lieutenant Governor for his consideration, and that of the Council, & certain recommendations were preferred, (which recommendations were approved of), there is nevertheless not one of those measures which has been carried out with that system of organization which is essential for the preservation of the people, & without which, in periods of epidemic pestilence, there can be no assurance to the public that its available resources will secure the greatest saving of human life, and that an inconsiderate, if not wilful expenditure of the Public Money will not occur.

I have also to observe that the ordinary powers granted for the preservation of the Public health in times of ordinary salubrity are quite inadequate for meeting the emergencies created by the spread of a mortal and devastating epidemic.

I have therefore to submit for the consideration of your Excellency that it would be expedient:

1st to receive the resignation of the present members of the Board of Health,
2nd to constitute a medical board whose function or duty it should be from time to time to recommend such measures as it might deem necessary for the Public Health and to assist the Board of Health with its Counsel and advise, but which should have nothing whatever to do with the responsibility of carrying out of such measures or with their financial details.

3rd to reconstitute the Board of Health with such members being placed upon it at as will carefully direct superintend and see to the due and efficient carrying of health measures who will watch over the expenditure created by such measures, the responsible for the same to the Governor in Council, and the Legislature.

4th to give to the Board of Health thus constituted similar powers to issue orders and directions as are given by the English Nuisances Removal and Contagious Diseases Prevention Act,[456] and amended Acts, when epidemic emergencies threaten the Mother Country.

5th Such powers are at present put in force by an order of the Privy Council are for a limited period, and are renewed, or not according to the exigency of the occasion.

Although in this colony there are, & must be, great difficulties in duly carrying out the measures necessary for the Public Health, more especially at the present time, I am convinced that the same happy results would follow their adoption in this Colony, as have followed wherever they have been fairly brought into operation, and duly executed.

I have to add that the medical members of the Board entirely agree with me in the view which I take as to the expediency of the changes proposed, & that last night they divided the Town and Island into districts so that a waste of time and labour might no longer take place, but that their services might be more equally and fully bestowed upon the numerous sufferers that still unhappily exist.

I have the honour to be… Hector Gavin. Med. Inspector W. I. C.

*From the Honourable Drs Kirkwood, Chipman and Duncome to His Excellency the Governor.*
*Nassau, November 16, 1852*

Sir, Having understood it to be your Excellency's intention to submit to the Executive Council the expediency of reconstituting the Board of Health, we the undersigned professional members of that Board beg to signify to your Excellency our entire readiness to resign our seats at the Board.

We have the honor to be & etc. & etc.

Drs. W. Kirkwood, H.N. Chipman, Frederick Duncome.

*From Dr Hector Gavin to the editor of* The Nassau Guardian
*February 5, 1853*

Sir, - I am induced to forward to you the accompanying Tables and communication because I deem them to be of essential importance to the well-being of the people of this colony in the event of a re-outbreak of epidemic cholera in the spring or autumn of this year, and because I believe them of the highest value to the West India colonies which may be attacked by cholera, as showing that with the materials existing in each colony, great progress may be made in saving the lives of the people, and more especially of the peasantry attacked by this terrible disease.

Having presented to the Governor in Council my views as to the measures to be employed to avert the serious ravages of cholera, I was empowered – through my seat at the Board of Health – to enter upon and superintend one of the most important of those which I recommended, namely a system of *House to House Visitation*, by paid visitors under my own instructions and directions.

It is unnecessary for me to enter upon the obstructive course pursued in regard to nearly all the other measures which were recommended, further than to observe that with the exception of the system of house-to-house visitation, and of Depots and printed instructions, a policy was pursued which was contrary to that which I deemed advisable for those public interests, with the consideration of which I was especially charged.

In thus characterizing the policy pursued, I do no more than I did in London with those Public Boards which acted upon a policy similar to that position here, and which policy there, as here, greatly tended to prevent that full measure of relief from premature death and suffering being applied to "the people," which science and experience had proved to be adequate for the purposes of view.

"*Salus populi suprema lex*" has been a law acknowledged by all civilized people from the time when Egyptian plagues first prevailed to the present; and I should be wanting in duty did I not state that all has not been done here that could have been done seeing that the inference would then be that with the means of the Colony a hand, the science of prevention of disease was only able to accomplish what had been accomplished here.

On the other hand, I am desirous that it should be known among the other West Indian Colonies that there is just reason for building hopes of comparative immunity from epidemic cholera, if their Governments will take in sufficient time, the steps known and proved to be necessary to, and capable of avoiding, comparative safety. A percentage, varying from 18 to 10 of the affected districts, need not perish if the necessary measures be promptly and advisedly taken.

It is a matter, therefore, of great congratulation that, although by no means all that could be, and ought to have been, accomplished was attained, so much at least was secured as may serve for a basis for action in future similar calamities here, or in the other West India Colonies.

The point to which I wish to draw your attention is the system of house to house visitation, as was applied in Nassau, New Providence, and in order to understand it, it will be necessary to cast a careful and observing glance over the accompanying Tables.

The visitation extended over a period of 72 days, and was conducted partly under my own superintendence, and partly under that of others. A staff, varying from 8 to 4 visitors, was employed at 30 shillings per week [approximately $233.00 today], each, whose chief business it was to pass from house, to house, searching out the existence of cases of cholera in the first stage, and distributing medicines and information, and preventing – by timely succour, the disease passing on to the more fully formed and consequently less curable stages of the disease.

It was essential that the system should be promptly put in action, because, from the records of the Registrars of deaths, and of the medical man, it appears that fully 20 per cent of those who had previously died of cholera in Nassau, had died without any medical aid whatever – the number of those who had been sick, and "ye visited not," was of course proportionate.

The town of Nassau was divided into five districts – 1. The East; 2. The West; 3. Bain's and Delancy Town; 4. Grant's Town; 5. The Town. This last district, on account of the parties who inhabit it being nearly all in a position of life which enabled them to pay for medical relief, was not put under visitation, and was moreover affected to but a very small extent by the epidemic.

From the tables it appears that an aggregate of not less than 1,817 cases of choleraic disease were discovered by the House-to-House Visitors during the period of visitation, which lasted 72 days, – that that of that number there were 1,616 cases of diarrhea, or simple looseness of the bowels, 159 cases of approaching cholera, or where cramps, spasms, severe, or white rice water purging, and vomiting present; 31 cases of advanced or developed cholera, and 11 corpses.

A careful inspection of this table will show that during the first week of the visitation, a very large number of cases of cholera in the 2nd and 3rd stages were discovered. The cases discovered being in the proportion of 100 cases of looseness, 14.5 of approaching cholera. During the next three weeks the aggregate number of cases of diarrhea amounted to about double that of the first week of the visitation, but the proportion of approaching cholera and cholera cases, in place of being 14.5 and five were only 7.3 and 2.3. This shows a marked reduction in the severe forms of the disease, arising from the milder cases of looseness being caught up and prevented passing on into the more fully formed stages of the disease.

It will be observed, that without any increase in the number of cases of diarrhea in the 5th week, the cases of advanced color increased alarmingly; thus, for every 100 cases of looseness discovered, they were 17.2 cases approaching cholera, and 4.5 cases of actual cholera, whilst more than a third of the total number of cops is discovered in that week.

This increase in the numbers affected by the disease mopped and increasing severity of it, shown in the increased mortality, as well as in the number of persons who were discovered to have died without medical aid, 11 persons who died between the 13th and the 20th of the month, both inclusive, six died without medical aid. The total number discovered by the visitors to have died without medical aid during the visitation amounts to 11. These facts prove that more active measures were urgently required to meet the disease, and my colleagues at the board cannot fail to recollect a renewed attempt to secure responsible medical officers to obey the Instructions to be issued by us, and the rebuff from the governor in Council which attended our efforts – a rebuff which led to my own resignation, and subsequently deprived the Board of the voluntary aid rendered by the medical men. But antecedent to this state of things, and a few days after my arrival from Harbour Island, it will also be within the recollection of my colleagues, that I availed myself of the discretionary power placed in my hands, and increased the number of Visitors, and the discipline established among them.

During the 6th week, with an increasing mortality doubling that of the previous weeks, the Visitors discovered nearly twice as many cases of looseness, while the number of cases of approaching cholera and cholera, which in the fifth week has been to every 100 cases of looseness 17.3 and 4.5, felt a six and 2.3.

The high mortality, however, the highest which had occurred in any 7 consecutive days from 25th November, showed that a number of persons were not brought under treatment until the disease and become so far developed as to be hopeless. This increase in the mortality was to be accounted for in two ways; first, by one of those sudden aggravations of the disease occurring, which frequently take place towards the end of an epidemic, like the flaring up of the flickering light of an expiring candle, – and secondly, by a diminution, or at least a not equally corresponding increase in the frequency and regularity of the visitation system.

I believe the first was the cause of the sudden increase in the extension severity of the disease. It is important, however, but it should be widely known that what is required to meet such sudden aggravations with success is increased frequency and discipline in the system of visitation.

It was for this reason that I brought to bear the whole force which the Board was empowered to employ for the reduction of mortality, and for the saving of lives of those seriously menaced. This additional force was the more necessary, from the Board (through the Governor in Council) having no Medical men to whom they could give order on the occasion. The districts of the

Visitors were diminished in size, and the visits were increased in frequency. Before this it was scarcely practicable for the Visitor to go over his whole district twice a day, – after this increase of the staff, and visitation of the districts, each affected district was visited 2 or 3 times a day, and each person whom the day previously was ill, was seen almost invariably before breakfast-time that morning, and again as circumstances demanded, in the course of the day.

Happy results are shown in the summaries of the seventh and eighth weeks. In these two weeks nearly one-third of the whole number of cases of diarrhea that were discovered well found, and very nearly a third of the whole number of cases approaching cholera with found, or found in these two weeks: – whereas, only two cases of cholera or 1/15th of the number of the cholera cases discovered were found, and no corpses. Moreover, the mortality in the 7th week 55.6 per cent and in the 8th week 78.6 per cent, as compared with the mortality of the sixth week.

The system of House-to-House visitation is thus sufficiently proved to have been adequate [for] the saving of human life, and therefore to be of paramount necessity in all places where cholera is existent.

I do not pretend for a moment that it was as sufficiently carried out as the visitation in the district of London which I had charge of in 1849. But, considering that the persons employed here as visitors were of an humble class in society, and (with the exception of one or two) were not of more than very ordinary degrees of intelligence, – whereas the parties employed in London were educated professional men, and advanced students of medicine, at from four to six guineas per week [up to $880 today], and were constantly supervised by Inspectors specially qualified in the work of prevention, – and comparing the results of the two visitations, I think there is still great reason to be satisfied, and that an assurance cannot be arrived at, that the system worked well, and saved the lives of very many persons who must otherwise have unavoidably perished.

Let it be remarked that of the whole number of cases discovered in the first stage of the disease, only 27 went on uncontrolled to the second stage, and that of 159 cases discovered in the second stage 147 were prevented passing on into fully developed cholera, whereas of the 31 cases discovered in the third stage, no less than 28 passed on into death.

In other words, 1 in 60 or 1.6 per cent of the cases in the first stage passed into the second stage; first in the 13 ½ or 7.5 percent of the cases in the second stage passed into the third, and 1 in 1.1 or 90.3 per cent in the third stage went on to death.

It is with much pleasure I append the testimony of the local medical practitioners to the efficiency of the system. Their unbiased evidence proves the advantages which one measure of safety alone has realised and I cannot but tend my cordial thanks and warm gratitude for the assistance which they rendered to me in carrying out, and thus demonstrating here, the value of the system of organized house to house visitation under qualified Inspectors.

Voluntarily and promptly, they gave succour where indicated by the visitors, and took charge of the advanced cases of the disease. It is infinitely to be regretted that their cooperation with the Board of Health could not, – notwithstanding all the necessities of the occasion, and all the efforts of the Board, be placed on a basis which would have rendered their services still more available for the saving of life and the alleviation of suffering, – for then they would have diminished the existent orphanage and widowhood, and prevented much distress.

I am, Sir, Your obedient Servant,
HECTOR GAVIN, M.D.,
Medical Inspector West India Colonies.
February 4th, 1853.

| Week | Visits | 1st stage | 2nd stage | 3rd stage | Corpses | Total | Deaths |
|---|---|---|---|---|---|---|---|
| 1 | 43 | 173 | 26 | 9 | 0 | 213 | 20 |
| 2 | 42 | 136 | 6 | 3 | 2 | 147 | 9 |
| 3 | 39 | 100 | 12 | 4 | 0 | 116 | 12 |
| 4 | 35 | 104 | 7 | 1 | 2 | 114 | 7 |
| 5 | 31 | 110 | 19 | 5 | 4 | 138 | 8 |
| 6 | 32 | 217 | 13 | 5 | 2 | 237 | 14 |
| 7 | 56 | 301 | 34 | 1 | 0 | 336 | 6 |
| 8 | 51 | 216 | 20 | 1 | 0 | 237 | 3 |
| 9 | 44 | 153 | 14 | 1 | 1 | 169 | 6 |
| 10 | 34 | 83 | 7 | 1 | 0 | 91 | 1 |
| Last 3 days | 15 | 18 | 1 | 0 | 0 | 19 | 1 |
| **Total** | **422** | **1611** | **159** | **31** | **11** | **1817** | **87** |

Summary of table published with Dr Gavin's letter dated February 4, 1853, showing cholera cases discovered by house-to-house visitors in New Providence from November 18, 1852 to January 29, 1853. *Source*: 'Cholera Cases Statistics Table'. *The Nassau Guardian*, February 5, 1853.

# Appendix 4

## *Cholera Expenses Presented to the Government*

### Harbour Island, December 1852–February 1853

| Amount Claimed | Pounds | Shillings |
|---|---|---|
| P. Higgs for house visiting at 30 shillings/wk | 1 | 10 |
| Joseph H. Cleare for 3 wks. visiting | 4 | 10 |
| Winer Bethel for 2 weeks visiting | 1 | 10 |
| W. Bethel for 1 week visiting | 1 | 10 |
| Joseph H. Cleare for 2 weeks visiting | 3 | 0 |
| Samuel Ingraham for 4 weeks medicine depot | 1 | 5 |
| Capt. John Bethel medicine depot and hospital steward | 2 | 18 |
| Mr. W. Cash for supplies to cholera hospital | 13 | 19 |
| Judith Roberts account | 0 | 18 |
| Mr. Sears for Elias Crofts, cholera hospital nurse at 12s. 6d. per diem | 7 | 17 |
| Mahaley Roberts, cholera hospital nurse | 24 | 15 |
| Joseph Saunders: bed and blanket for the cholera hospital per Dr. Eneas | 0 | 12 |
| Samuel Ingraham: keeping cholera depot 3 weeks | 0 | 18 |
| J. H. Johnson account | 0 | 14 |
| Dr. Wendall's bills for medicines | 20 | 0 |
| Dr. Eneas for medicines | 26 | 6 |
| Dr. Eneas for bread, fowls, food for the hospital, other sundries, porterage | 5 | 0 |
| W. H. Sears account for food for poor | 0 | 19 |
| **Total** | **119** | **15** |

# House of Assembly Appropriations Bill, 1853

| Amount Approved for Payment | Pounds | Shillings | Pence |
|---|---|---|---|
| To Estate of Dr. Wendall for attendance on the poor afflicted with cholera at Harbour Island 57 days at £2.2s | 119 | 14 | 0 |
| To Dr. Eneas for like services 68 days at £2.2s | 142 | 16 | 0 |
| Mr. William A. Smith for three weeks attendance at 12s.6d and medicines | 13 | 2 | 6 |
| Mrs. Sarah Lowe, for rent of premises for Hospital at Harbour Island, furniture damaged, repairing and painting | 20 | 16 | 8 |
| Dr Kirkwood for 8 days attendance on the poor at Nassau at £2.2s | 16 | 16 | 0 |
| Dr Chipman for 8 days attendance on the poor at Nassau at £2.2s | 16 | 16 | 0 |
| Dr Duncome for 8 days attendance on the poor at Nassau at £2.2s | 16 | 16 | 0 |
| Mr Black for 8 days attendance on the poor at Nassau at £2.2s | 16 | 16 | 0 |
| Dr Kirkwood for medicines supplied to the poor at Nassau and Out-islands | 181 | 15 | 0 |
| Apothecaries' Hall for medicines supplied to the poor at Nassau and Out-islands | 216 | 6 | 6 |
| Mr Plackledge, Governor's Harbour, for attendance night and day and administering medicines 42 days at 12s.6d per day | 26 | 5 | 0 |
| Messrs. Avery Bethel and Charles Bethel (employed by the Local Board of Health) for attending and visiting the sick 22 days each at 4s.2d | 9 | 3 | 4 |
| Messrs Thomas Griffin and Kersey Stirrup house-to-house Visitors, 22 days at 2s.1d per day | 4 | 11 | 8 |
| Account for sundry expenses of the Board on account of cholera patients at Governor's Harbour | 22 | 15 | 6 |
| Richard Knowles, Tarpum Bay, for digging graves | 2 | 1 | 8 |
| Daniel Evans, for attendance and administering medicines | 3 | 0 | 0 |
| Sarah Ann Culmer, for attendance and administering medicines | 3 | 0 | 0 |
| Rina McKenzie, for attendance and administering medicines | 3 | 0 | 0 |
| Dr Samuel Clutsam, for three weeks' attendance on the poor at Rock Sound, being the period for which he was employed at £2.2s | 44 | 2 | 0 |
| Dr Samuel Clutsam, for his passage to Nassau | 2 | 1 | 8 |
| John A. Cooper and others at Exuma, making coffins, digging graves, attending and visiting the sick, and burying 13 persons who died of cholera (4 in coffins, 9 sewn in mats – per petition submitted March 17, 1853) | 26 | 5 | 0 |
| Charles Bethel, Eleuthera, for amount paid by him for conveying cholera supplies from Nassau to Eleuthera | 2 | 1 | 8 |
| Robert Dorritie, for 1,390 cabbages thrown away by order of the Health Officer, cost $97.30 | 20 | 5 | 5 |
| James Ross, Sexton of St. Matthew's for this sum paid by him to William Minus as an assistant during the prevalence of cholera, 5 weeks at 9s.4d | 2 | 6 | 10 |
| James Ross for digging six graves for persons who died of cholera | 1 | 9 | 2 |
| James Ross for extra services during the prevalence of cholera | 5 | 0 | 0 |
| **Total** | **942** | **3** | **7** |

*Source*: 'Proceedings of the Hon. House of Assembly, Wednesday Afternoon 6th April, 1853'. *The Nassau Guardian*, April 9, 1853. 'Proceedings of the Hon. House of Assembly, Report of the Select Committee for Unliquidated Claims Arising Out of the Recent Choleraic Epidemic'. *The Nassau Guardian*, April 16, 1853.

# Appendix 5

## *Number of Deaths in The Bahamas, 1848–1855*

*Source*: The Bahamas Blue Book Reports for 1848–1855.
Bahamas Department of Archives.

| **Island** | **1847** | **1848** | **1849** | **1850** | **1851** | **1852** | **1853** | **1854** | **1855** |
|---|---|---|---|---|---|---|---|---|---|
| New Providence | 184 | 59 | 57 | - | 231 | 924 | 255 | 202 | 160 |
| Harbour Island | 26 | 34 | 25 | - | 54 | 217 | 43 | 49 | 20 |
| Eleuthera | | | | | 88 | 155 | 62 | 39 | 67 |
| Rum Cay | 2 | - | 4 | | 19 | 6 | 25 | 15 | 9 |
| Crooked Island | 10 | - | - | | 6 | 9 | 13 | 20 | 12 |
| San Salvador | | | | | 33 | 26 | 25 | 36 | 20 |
| Exuma | - | 30 | 10 | | 34 | 42 | 22 | 24 | 27 |
| Long Island | | | | | 22 | 23 | 17 | 8 | 12 |
| Abaco | - | 4 | 11 | | 37 | 148 | 27 | 34 | 42 |
| Ragged Island | - | 5 | 0 | | 9 | 45 | 3 | 6 | 0 |
| Andros | | | | | 15 | 20 | 8 | 11 | 8 |
| Grand Bahama | | | | | 16 | 26 | 11 | 16 | 8 |
| Berry Island | | | | | 4 | 0 | 5 | 6 | 3 |
| Bimini | | | | | 2 | 12 | 2 | 5 | 2 |
| Watlings Island | | | | | - | 13/3 | 5 | 4 | 9 |
| Inagua and Mayaguana | | | | | - | 0 | 17 | 11 | 28 |
| **Total deaths*** | **222** | **129** | **107** | **-** | **576** | **1656** | **540** | **499** | **427** |
| **Population** | | | | | **27601** | | | | |
| **Crude death rate**** | **-** | **-** | **-** | **-** | **20.9** | **62.5** | **19.6** | **18.0** | **15.4** |

*Pre-1851 data incomplete

** Approximation

# Appendix 6

## *Executive Council Meetings: Attendees Listed in the Roll from Minutes, September–November 1852*

The governor's decisions were formulated on the advice, but not necessarily the consent, of the Executive Council, an eight or nine-member body of prominent White residents. The colonial secretary, attorney general and the receiver-general (treasurer) were *ex-officio* members.

**September 28, 1852**
His Honour the Lieutenant Governor
George C. Anderson (Attorney General)
William Vesey Munnings (Provost Marshal)
Felix MacCarthy (Police Magistrate)
John G. Anderson (Receiver General)
Robert A. Thomson

**October 2, 1852**
The Lieutenant Governor
George C. Anderson
Thomas Martin Mathews
William Vesey Munnings
Robert Thomson
Felix MacCarthy
J. G. Anderson

**October 5, 1852**
The Lieutenant Governor
Attorney General
Receiver General
Matthews
William V. Munnings
Robert Thomson

**October 9, 1852**
The Lieutenant Governor
Attorney General
William Webb (1791–1867): retired
Collector of Customs
T. M. Mathews
William V. Munnings
F. MacCarthy
J. G. Anderson

**October 12, 1852**
The Lieutenant Governor
Attorney General
Receiver General
William Webb
William Vesey Munnings
Robert Thomson
Felix MacCarthy

**October 13, 1852**
The Lieutenant Governor
Attorney General
Receiver General
William V. Munnings
Robert Thomson
Felix MacCarthy
Thomas Martin Mathews

**October 15, 1852**
The Lieutenant Governor
Attorney General
William Webb
Thomas Martin Mathews
Robert Thomson
Receiver General
Felix MacCarthy
William V. Munnings

**October 26, 1852**
The Lieutenant Governor
Attorney General
Receiver General
William Webb
William V. Munnings
T. M. Mathews
Felix MacCarthy
Robert Thomson

**November 2, 1852**
The Lieutenant Governor
George C. Anderson
John G. Anderson
Thomas Martin Mathews
William Webb
William Vesey Munnings
R. Thomson

**November 10, 1852**
His Excellency the Governor
Colonial Secretary
George C. Anderson
William Webb
John G. Anderson
Felix MacCarthy
William Vesey Munnings

**November 16, 1852**
His Excellency the Governor
Colonial Secretary
George C. Anderson
William Webb
John G. Anderson
Felix MacCarthy
William Vesey Munnings

**22 November 1852**
His Excellency the Governor
Colonial Secretary
G. C. Anderson
William Webb
John G. Anderson
Felix MacCarthy
Robert Thomson
Thomas Martin Mathews
William Vesey Munnings

# Appendix 7

## Sailing Ships

- The *Pedraza*, built in Philadelphia in 1833, weighed 139 tons and had dimensions of 77' x 23' x 9'. She had one deck, two square-rigged masts, a square stern and a woman-bust figurehead. She was previously registered on July 10, 1847 at New York City, and temporarily registered on June 23, 1851. The owners were Lucas B. Terry (one-third) and John F. Bacon (two-thirds) of New York City. Her master was Robert Dorritie of New York City. The vessel was condemned as being unseaworthy at the port of Nassau,[i] shortly after her temporary registration in 1851, when she was eighteen years old. The normal life expectancy for a similar vessel would be twenty to twenty-five years. The long-distance blue-water voyages that she made may have accelerated her ageing; however, it is likely that the cholera epidemic finished her off. Who would want to crew this worn-out ship after all of the cholera deaths aboard?

- Other brigs or brigantines include the *Edinburgh*, *Baltic*, *Hope*, *Victoria* and *Wild Pigeon*, all sailing vessels with two square-rigged masts. They were fast and manoeuvrable but required a relatively large crew and were difficult to sail into the wind. Perhaps the most famous brig was the HMS *Beagle*, in which Charles Darwin sailed around the world from 1831 to 1836.

- A barque is a sailing ship typically with three masts, in which the foremast and mainmast are square-rigged and the mizzenmast is rigged fore and aft. Examples include the *Ovando*, *Rio* and *William and Mary*.

- A schooner is a two-masted sailing vessel, fore- and aft-rigged on both masts. They are relatively easy to handle in confined waters and require a relatively smaller crew. Examples include the *Iowa*, the *Reform,* which brought cholera to New Providence, *Lelia*, the *Clyde*, *Atlantic* and *Violin*.

- A screw steamer is a sailing vessel with a steam engine for main or supplemental power and using a propeller as opposed to a paddle to propel it through the water. Examples include the *Esk* and *Conway*.

- Royal Mail Steam Ship *La Plata*. Commissioned 1852. Gross tons 2,292. Length 285 feet. A fast paddle steamer that could average over 12 knots. She transported the governor and his family from Southampton to St. Thomas on his return from vacation. Yellow fever ravaged the ship during her return to

England. It killed nine persons, including her commander and on arrival at Southampton, some twenty-one were seriously ill, including the doctor. *La Plata* was quarantined and after it was learned that the *Esk*, which had also departed St. Thomas and had yellow fever aboard, had not been quarantined, an inquiry was opened. A series of sharp letters were exchanged between Sir William Pym, the Superintendent-General of Quarantine and Hector Gavin, moderated the General Board of Health. *La Plata* continued service until November 18, 1867, when she was destroyed, with the loss of her crew, by the tsunami that followed the Virgin Islands earthquake.

# Appendix 8

## *New Providence Asylum Annual Expenses, 1850*

| **Salary** | **Pounds** | **Shillings** | **Equivalent in 2023 (£)** |
|---|---|---|---|
| Asylum superintendent | 208 | 6 | 23,422 |
| Asylum physician | 94 | 11 | 10,584 |
| Asylum chaplain | 25 | 0 | 2,815 |
| Matron | 25 | 0 | 2,815 |
| Attendants | 75 | 0 | 8,445 |
| Asylum provisions | 680 | 0 | 76,572 |
| Dispensary keeper | 20 | 0 | 2,252 |
| Dispensary physician | 60 | 0 | 6,756 |
| African Hospital physician | 40 | 0 | 4,614 |

# Appendix 9

*Board of Health Act 1850 (Excerpt)*

The Board of Health appointed under the Act 13th Victoria Chapter 21, have directed the publication of the following sections of the said Act for the information of the Public:

**Section IX.** And whereas, causes of sickness may arise from allowing weeds to grow, filth to accumulate or stagnant water to lie, or offensive substances to be brought within the several towns of the colony: Be it enacted that if the proprietor or occupier of any lot of land situate within the limits of the town of Nassau and suburbs thereof, extending east to Church street, west to the eastern boundary of the Ordnance Ground surrounding Fort Charlotte, and south to Grant's Town or any other town within these Islands, shall permit or suffer weeds to grow in such lot or shall permit any description of filth or rubbish to accumulate therein, or any stagnant water to be and remain therein and shall not remove the same within a reasonable time … [shall upon conviction be liable to a] sum not exceeding ten pounds, over and above the expense incurred in the removal or abatement of the nuisance.

**Section X.** And Whereas it would tend much to the health of towns if the depth of Privies were regulated: Be it enacted that every privy situate and being within any town in this Colony of less depth than six feet, shall be deemed, held and taken to be a public nuisance, and the owner thereof or in the absence of the owner from the Colony, the person having charge of the land on which such Privy is situated, shall be liable to be proceeded against as and for a public nuisance, if on notice thereof being given to him or her, such nuisance is not forthwith abated; such notice to be given by the Inspector or Chief Officer of Police, or by any Constable acting under the orders of such Inspector, or Chief Officer of Police, when the nuisance complained of exists in the Island of New Providence; and by any Constable acting under the orders of a Justice of the Peace, where the nuisance complained of exists on an out Island of the Government.

*Source*: Nassau, June 14, 1850, published in the *Bahama Herald*, June 26, 1850.

# Appendix 10

## *Health Patterns among Creole Slaves, 1834*

*Source:* 'Slave Register 1834', in Saunders, Gail. *Slavery in The Bahamas, 1648–1838.* D. G. Saunders, 1985.

| Age | 0–10 | 11–15 | 16–25 | 26–29 | 30–39 | 40–49 | 50–59 | 60–69 | 70–79 | 80+ | Total |
|---|---|---|---|---|---|---|---|---|---|---|---|
| Effective | 1,191 | 1,126 | 1,787 | 674 | 1,091 | 552 | 278 | 122 | 28 | 7 | 6,851 |
| Non-effective | 2,077 | 8 | 14 | 7 | 9 | 7 | 12 | 29 | 29 | 6 | 2,198 |
| Bodily disease | 0 | 0 | 4 | 5 | 6 | 1 | 3 | 4 | 2 | 1 | 26 |
| Rupture | 0 | 0 | 0 | 0 | 3 | 0 | 2 | 3 | 1 | 0 | 9 |
| Lameness | 0 | 1 | 2 | 3 | 1 | 5 | 0 | 0 | 0 | 0 | 12 |
| Deaf-dumb | | | 1 | | 1 | | | | | | 2 |
| Rheumatism | | | | | 1 | | | | | | 1 |
| Ulcerated leg | | | 1 | | 2 | 2 | 3 | | 1 | | 9 |
| Mental illness | | | | | 1 | | | 1 | | | 2 |
| Blindness | | | | | | | 2 | | | | 2 |
| Scrofula* | | | 1 | | | | | | | | 1 |
| Phthisis** | | | | | | 2 | 1 | | | | 3 |
| Leprosy | | | | | 1 | | | | | | 1 |
| Dysentery | | | | | | | | | | | - |
| Spine infection | | 1 | | | | | | | | | 1 |
| Asthma | | | 1 | | | | | | | | 1 |
| Hysteric fits | | | 2 | 1 | | | | | | | 3 |
| Elephantiasis | | | | | | 1 | | | | | 1 |
| Too young | 2,074 | | | | | | | | | | 2,074 |
| Old age | | | | | | | 6 | 20 | 25 | 5 | 56 |

*Scrofula: tuberculosis of the lymph glands of the neck; **phthisis: tuberculosis of the lung.

# Appendix 11

## *Returns of Births and Deaths, January 1–June 30, 1852*

*Source:* 'New Providence Board of Health'. *The Nassau Guardian,* September 18, 1852.

| Islands | Births | Deaths | Whooping cough | Dropsy | Fever | Dysentery | Lockjaw | Teething | Consumption | Violence | Other |
|---|---|---|---|---|---|---|---|---|---|---|---|
| NP | 209 | 112 | 2 | 3 | 18 | 6 | 3 | 5 | 16 | 4 | 54 |
| Harbour Is. | 61 | 17 | 0 | 0 | 7 | 1 | 0 | 0 | 2 | 2 | 7 |
| Eleuthera | 85 | 32 | 0 | 1 | 5 | 8 | 6 | 0 | 4 | 0 | 8 |
| San Sal. | 42 | 6 | 0 | 0 | 3 | 0 | 0 | 0 | 0 | 0 | 3 |
| Exumas | 41 | 6 | 0 | 0 | 1 | 0 | 1 | 0 | 0 | 1 | 1 |
| Crooked Is. | 27 | 5 | 0 | 0 | 3 | 0 | 0 | 0 | 0 | 0 | 2 |
| Long Is . | 35 | 13 | 0 | 3 | 3 | 0 | 0 | 0 | 1 | 0 | 6 |
| Andros | 16 | 5 | 0 | 0 | 0 | 0 | 0 | 0 | 1 | 2 | 2 |
| Grand Bah. | 13 | 13 | 0 | 0 | 0 | 0 | 0 | 0 | 0 | 2 | 11 |
| Watlings Is. | 8 | 2 | 0 | 1 | 0 | 0 | 0 | 0 | 0 | 0 | 1 |
| Rum Cay | 17 | 5 | 0 | 0 | 0 | 1 | 2 | 0 | 0 | 0 | 2 |
| Inagua | 0 | 0 | 0 | 0 | 0 | 0 | 0 | 0 | 0 | 0 | 0 |
| Abaco | 34 | 30 | 0 | 0 | 10 | 1 | 0 | 0 | 1 | 9 | 9 |
| Ragged Is. | 10 | 5 | 0 | 0 | 0 | 1 | 0 | 0 | 0 | 1 | 3 |
| Acklins | 8 | 1 | 0 | 0 | 0 | 0 | 0 | 0 | 0 | 0 | 1 |
| Bimini | 6 | 0 | 0 | 0 | 0 | 0 | 0 | 0 | 0 | 0 | 0 |
| Berry Is. | 0 | 0 | 0 | 0 | 0 | 0 | 0 | 0 | 0 | 0 | 0 |
| **Total** | **612** | **252** | **2** | **8** | **50** | **18** | **12** | **5** | **25** | **19** | **112** |

# Appendix 12

## *Population of The Bahamas, 1838–2010*

*Source:* Bahamas Department of Statistics.

| Census | Population | Increase | Increase (%) | Annual Increase | Annual Growth |
|---|---|---|---|---|---|
| **1838** | 21,794 | - | - | - | - |
| **1845** | 26,491 | 4,697 | 21.55 | 671 | 3.1 |
| **1851** | 27,519 | 1,028 | 3.88 | 171 | 0.6 |
| **1861** | 35,487 | 7,668 | 28.95 | 797 | 2.9 |
| **1871** | 39,162 | 3,675 | 10.36 | 367 | 1.0 |
| **1881** | 43,521 | 4,359 | 11.13 | 436 | 1.1 |
| **1891** | 47,565 | 4,044 | 9.29 | 404 | 0.9 |
| **1901** | 53,735 | 6,170 | 12.97 | 617 | 1.3 |
| **1911** | 55,944 | 2,209 | 4.11 | 221 | 0.4 |
| **1921** | 53,031 | -2,913 | -5.21 | -291 | -0.6 |
| **1931** | 59,828 | 6,797 | 12.82 | 680 | 1.2 |
| **1943** | 68,846 | 9,018 | 15.07 | 751 | 1.2 |
| **1953** | 84,841 | 15,995 | 23.23 | 1,599 | 2.0 |
| **1963** | 130,220 | 45,379 | 53.49 | 4,538 | 4.4 |
| **1970** | 168,812 | 38,592 | 29.64 | 5,513 | 3.8 |
| **1980** | 209,505 | 40,693 | 24.11 | 4,069 | 2.2 |
| **1990** | 255,049 | 45,544 | 21.74 | 4,554 | 2.0 |
| **2000** | 303,611 | 48,562 | 19.04 | 4,856 | 1.8 |
| **2010** | 351,461 | 47,850 | 15.8 | 4,785 | 1.6 |

# Appendix 13

## *Population of The Bahamas by Island, 1851*

*Source:* Bahamas Department of Archives.

| **Island** | **Population** |
|---|---|
| New Providence | 8,159 |
| Eleuthera | 4,610 |
| Exuma | 2,027 |
| Abaco | 2,011 |
| Harbour Island | 1,840 |
| Cat Island (St Salvador) | 1,828 |
| Long Island | 1,477 |
| Crooked Island, Long Cay and Acklins | 1,092 |
| Andros | 1,030 |
| Grand Bahama | 922 |
| Rum Cay | 858 |
| Mayaguana and Inagua | 530 |
| Watlings (San Salvador) | 384 |
| Ragged Island | 347 |
| Berry Islands | 336 |
| Bimini | 150 |
| **Total** | **27,601** |

# Appendix 14

## *Epidemic Statistics*

Abstract of returns from the Board of Health of the number of cases of cholera and deaths. *Source: The Nassau Guardian,* October 2, 16, 23 and 27, November 3, 6, 17, 24 and 27, December 1, 1852.

| Date (1852) | Cases | Deaths |
|---|---|---|
| September 21 | 19 | 2 |
| September 22 | 10 | 0 |
| September 23 | 25 | 6 |
| September 24 | 12 | 4 |
| September 25 | 9 | 5 |
| September 26 | 14 | 6 |
| September 27 | 22 | 9 |
| September 28 | 6 | 2 |
| September 29 and 30 | 57 | 18 |
| **Total** | **174** | **52** |

| Date (1852) | Cases | Deaths |
|---|---|---|
| October 1 | 33 | 2 |
| October 2 | 28 | 9 |
| October 3 | 42 | 7 |
| October 4 | 36 | 3 |
| October 5 | 13 | 5 |
| October 6 | 21 | 5 |
| October 7 | 13 | 5 |
| October 8 | 33 | 6 |
| October 9 | 29 | 4 |
| October 10 | - | - |
| October 11 | 73 | 26 |
| October 12 | 34 | 6 |
| October 13 | 30 | 6 |
| October 14 | 48 | 15 |
| October 15 | 46 | 17 |
| October 16 | 30 | 53 |
| October 17 | 30 | 17 |
| October 18 | 32 | 18 |
| October 19 | 42 | 10 |
| October 20 | 55 | 16 |
| October 21 | 37 | 19 |
| October 22 | 54 | 12 |
| October 23 | 61 | 13 |
| October 24 | 19 | 7 |
| October 25 | 27 | 7 |
| October 26 | 26 | 6 |
| October 27 | 23 | 6 |
| October 28 | 35 | 13 |
| October 29 | 32 | 5 |
| October 30 | 23 | 11 |
| October 31 | 14 | 4 |
| **Total** | **771** | **287** |

| Date (1852) | Cases | Deaths | Non-cholera deaths |
|---|---|---|---|
| November 1 | 26 | 3 | |
| November 2 | 28 | 8 | |
| November 3 | 27 | 10 | |
| November 4 | 22 | 6 | |
| November 5 | 23 | 5 | |
| November 6 | 12 | 3 | |
| November 7 | 16 | 4 | |
| November 8 | 23 | 1 | |
| November 9 | 22 | 4 | |
| November 10 | 25 | 14 | |
| November 11 | 19 | 9 | |
| November 12 | 7 | 1 | |
| November 13 | 7 | 0 | |
| November 14 | 5 | 0 | |
| November 15 | 5 | 0 | |
| November 16 | 6 | 0 | |
| November 17 | 5 | 1 | |
| November 18 | 9 | 0 | |
| November 19 | 5 | 0 | |
| November 20 | - | 3 | 1 |
| November 21 | - | 3 | 0 |
| November 22 | - | 3 | 1 |
| November 23 | - | 2 | 2 |
| November 24 | - | 1 | 0 |
| November 25 | - | 1 | 1 |
| November 26 | - | 2 | 0 |
| **Total** | 292 | 84 | 5 |

Cholera at Fresh Creek, Andros, *Source:* 'Board of Health Returns'. *The Nassau Guardian,* November 17, 1852.

| Date 1852 | Cases | Deaths |
|---|---|---|
| October 12 | 2 | 0 |
| October 19 | 1 | 0 |
| October 20 | 1 | 1 |
| October 21 | 1 | 0 |
| October 22 | 2 | 1 |
| October 23 | 1 | 1 |
| October 24 | 1 | 0 |
| October 25 | 2 | 0 |
| October 26 | 2 | 2 |
| October 27 | 1 | 0 |
| October 28 | 2 | 0 |
| Total deaths | 16 | 5 |

# Appendix 15

## *Deaths and Cumulative Mortality from Cholera in New Providence, September–November 1852*

Abstract of returns from the Board of Health of the number of cases of cholera and deaths. *Source: The Nassau Guardian,* October 2, 16, 23 and 27, November 3, 6, 17, 24 and 27, December 1, 1852.

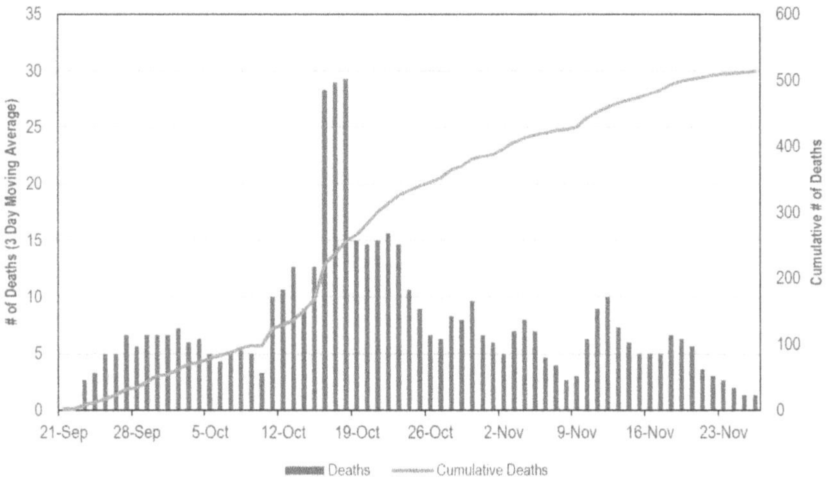

# Appendix 16

## *'How to Avoid Fever, Consumption or Cholera: Papers on Sanitation' (Excerpt)*

*Source*: 'How to Avoid Fever, Consumption or Cholera: Papers on Sanitation by the Hon. W. Kirkwood MD MLC, Hon. G.T.R. Kemp MD MEC, J. B. Albury MD, W. Robinson LRCSI and Hon W. M. G. Maclure MD MLC. With an Introduction by His Excellency the Governor', 1884. CO 23/225, Bahamas Department of Archives.

### Booklet Introduction by Governor Blake

The following papers on simple rules for the preservation of health were read for rent by the five medical gentlemen living in Nassau at meetings convened by me, and held in the various districts of the town, to consider the best means by which the advance of disease can be checked, and the effects minimized of any epidemic that may unfortunately visit the islands of this colony.

The primary reason for this action was the alarming reports of the reappearance of cholera in Europe, and the possibility that it may within a year or so extend to America and find its way to the Bahamas. I found on inquiry that the last epidemic of cholera in 1852 carried off one tenth of the inhabitants of Grants Town and the Eastern District of Nassau that the violence of the scourge of these districts was in consequence of the unsanitary condition of the houses and surroundings, and, as there has been no improvement made in that condition since 1852, there is the greatest reason to fear that if something be not done to render the houses, and enclosures, and mode of living more healthy, any return of cholera would probably sweep away as many people as were destroyed by the last epidemic.

But I found further, that putting aside any question of the appearance of an epidemic of cholera or other disease, the same precautions that are found in other countries to be effectual in checking the progress of these epidemics are equally effective as preventing the occurrence of the more ordinary diseases, in so much that the average duration of life has been sensibly increased.

It was for the purpose of laying these facts before the public, and inviting their assistance in the matter that the meetings were convened by me, and I have every reason to be satisfied with the success that has so far attended the movement. Recognizing the fact that without the hearty and persevering cooperation of the people themselves no permanent improvement in their condition can be affected, I have suggested to the various divisions into which Nassau has been divided for the purpose, that they should each elect a local committee of five members, who would act as a local volunteer sanitary board, endeavoring to induce their neighbors to adopt the sanitary measures which were found necessary, and if persuasion failed, and bringing the names of the defaulters under the notice of the Board of Health. The people have met, and elected these local committees, which cannot fail to bring about a great and permanent improvement in the comfort and the health of the population.

So much for what has been done, and is being done in Nassau. But New Providence is only one of the many islands of the Bahamas, and I am anxious that the inhabitants of every portion of the Colony shall have an opportunity of studying the scientific lesson so generously placed before the Nassau people by the five medical gentlemen already named, and I'm adopting similar measures as a precaution against sickness. I therefore commend to the people of the out-islands the views expressed in this pamphlet by those gentlemen, and earnestly advocate the appointment of local volunteer boards of health at each out-settlement. These boards I wish to have elected by the house-holders, and I trust that by their example and exertions we may have the happiness of seeing greater evidence of comfort in and about the dwellings, and of finding a considerable decrease in the number of deaths from preventable causes.

The result of the medical testimony is, shortly, that overcrowding at night, impure water, rank vegetation, and decaying animal or vegetable matter about your houses are all potent causes of disease and death; while good ventilation, pure water, well weeded gardens, and properly arranged cesspools, on the simple dry earth system, will secure decency, comfort, and the unspeakable blessing of health. Should any inhabitant desire more detailed information on any matter of sanitation, an application to the Board of Health at Nassau will receive attention.

Having now brought this question before the inhabitants of the out-islands, I look without misgiving for the same evidence of self-help that is being given in Nassau, by the formation of the volunteer committees; and I fervently trust that should any epidemic disease be carried to these shores, it may find us prepared to face it with the confidence of men who, having taken timely precautions in their houses and surroundings, await its approach with courage and fortitude.

Henry W. Blake, Governor. Government House, Nassau, N.P. 19th September, 1884.

# Chapter notes

## Notes to Chapter 1

1 Farre, Frederick J. 'Cholera in The Bahamas'. *Medical Times and Gazette 6* (1853): 300–301.
2 Rosenberg, Charles E. *The Cholera Years: The United States in 1832, 1849 and 1866.* University of Chicago Press, 1962.
3 Exodus 8: swarms of frogs and insects preceded the plague of sickness.
4 Gray, H., M. Storr, R. Roberts & P. Johnson. *Health Care Reform: Policy Content and Process in the Caribbean: Study No 1: The Historical Development of the Health System in the Bahamas.* London School of Hygiene and Tropical Medicine, 2001.
5 The Medical Practitioners Act. Statute Law of The Bahama Islands, May 29, 1906.
6 Efforts to remove mercury from households have caused a disappearance of the once-popular antiseptic mercurochrome. Digital thermometers have replaced the old glass-and-mercury sticks. Today, most mercury poisoning comes from consuming fish caught in polluted water.
7 McCormack, Jeffrey, K. Maier & P. B. Wallens. *Bush Medicine of the Bahamas: A Cross-Cultural Perspective from San Salvador Island including Pharmacology and Oral Histories.* JHM Designs Publications, 2011: 4–9.
8 Analysis of Peter Solomon Townsend's diary: Kenny, E. 'Fictional Space and Taxonomies of Race in The Bahamas: Mapping American Identity in the Early Republic'. *Journal of Transatlantic Studies* 14(2) (2016): 139–151.
9 The incident occurred on C. R. Nesbitt's estate near Fort Montagu. The girl and her parents, who lived on the estate, were not named, so they would have been caretakers and likely former slaves. 'Editorial'. *The Nassau Guardian,* 19 December 1849.
10 Moseley, Mary. *The Bahamas Handbook 1926.* The Nassau Guardian, 1926: 43.
11 Lewis Grant, governor of The Bahamas from 1821 to 1829, died suddenly of a heart attack in 1852 while riding in an omnibus in London. 'Death of General Sir Lewis Grant KCH. Editorial'. *The Nassau Guardian,* March 13, 1852.
12 Saunders, Gail. *Bahamian Society after Emancipation.* MacMillan Caribbean, 2003.
13 'House of Assembly Proceedings'. *The Nassau Guardian,* March 2, 1850.
14 'Editorial'. *The Nassau Guardian,* March 30, 1850.
15 'Editorial'. *Bahama Herald,* April 2, 1850.
16 'Statement of Loss of Property Sustained in the Southern Suburbs of the Island of New Providence, Including Grant's Town, Delancy's Town and Bain's Town'. *Bahama Herald,* April 5, 1850.
17 'List of Appointments to Stipendiary Offices during the Administration of Ex-Governor Mathew: Natives or Colonists'. *The Nassau Guardian,* September 22, 1849.
18 'Letter to the Editor'. *Bahama Herald,* April 16, 1850.
19 'Deadly Tornado'. *Bahama Herald,* April 2 and April 19, 1850.
20 'Statement of Property Destroyed'. *The Nassau Guardian,* April 13, 1850.

21 'Government Notice'. *The Nassau Guardian,* April 20, 1850.
22 'Government Notice: Return of Births and Deaths for the Half-Year Ending the 30th June 1852'. *The Nassau Guardian,* September 18, 1852.
23 'Teething as a Cause of Death: A Historical Review'. *The Western Journal of Medicine,* 155 (December 1991): 658–659.
24 Whooping cough has not been seen in The Bahamas for many years, thanks to an effective immunisation programme. However, in the year 2020, Florida saw 200 cases. Florida Department of Health, 'Pertussis (Whooping Cough)', www.floridahealth.gov/diseases-and-conditions/vaccine-preventable-disease/pertussis/index.html, retrieved August 15, 2021.
25 'Government Notice: Return of Births and Deaths for the Half-Year Ending the 30th June 1852'. *The Nassau Guardian,* September 18, 1852.
26 Dahl-Regis, Merceline. *Annual Report of the Chief Medical Officer.* Ministry of Health, Commonwealth of The Bahamas, 2000.
27 'Statistical Returns for the Alexandria Wards'. Bahamas General Hospital, 1925.
28 The United States saw hundreds of thousands of cases every year and its mortality rate of 33 per cent caused the government in 1914 to establish the Spartanburg Pellagra Hospital in South Carolina to study and treat pellagra. Kiple, K. 'Pellagra'. The Cambridge World History of Human Disease. Cambridge University Press, 1993.
29 'Letter to the Editor'. *Bahama Herald.* October 16, 1852.
30 Here began the iconography of Over-the-Hill. In *Love and Responsibility: The Dawn Davis Collection* (2012), art historian Dr Erica James notes how these images sanitised their subject – the social narrative suppressed for the picturesque.
31 'Editorial'. *Bahama Herald,* March 5, 1851.
32 In July 1852, the Executive Council approved Chipman's request for permission to charge fees when visiting sailors were admitted to the Asylum, prompted by cases like the *Atlantic,* a vessel which departed Maine for Puerto Rico in February 1851 and ran into a storm. She reached New Providence with her sailors seriously ill. Chipman cared for them, an assignment above and beyond his normal responsibilities, for no extra pay ('Shipping Intelligence'. *Bahama Herald,* February 26, 1851).
33 'Hon. Dr William Kirkwood Obituary'. *The Nassau Guardian,* December 12, 1888.
34 The University of Pennsylvania was founded in 1765, ahead of Harvard (1782) and Dartmouth (1797).
35 Only in the twentieth century did medical education in America move from the lecture room to the hospital bedside. Bliss, Michael. *William Osler: A Life in Medicine.* Oxford University Press, 1999.
36 Moseley Moss, Valeria. *Reminiscing: Memories of Old Nassau.* R. G. Lightbourn, 1999: 106, 111.
37 In 1849, 85 per cent of the £30,776 that the colony realised from exports came from just two items: salt (52 per cent) and pineapples (33 per cent). The Bahamas Blue Book Report for 1849.
38 In March 1851, the Executive Council summoned Kirkwood to explain his company's plan to build a tramway in Matthew Town. Wind of the plan had reached residents and triggered a protest. Executive Council Minutes, March 3, 1851.
39 In the 1890s, the New Providence Asylum became the Bahamas General Hospital (BGH). A new BGH was built on the same site in 1952, which, three years after it opened, was renamed the Princess Margaret Hospital.
40 'Dr Frederick Duncombe Obituary'. *The Nassau Guardian,* March 25, 1882.
41 In 1849, Christ Church Sunday School moved to a new hall that had been built in part by a substantial donation from Dr Duncome. He continued as its superintendent for thirty years.
42 'Sudden Death. Editorial'. *Bahama Herald,* January 11, 1851.
43 The Centers for Disease Control identifies several natural sources of cyanide poisoning

hazard (see CDC. 'Cyanide: Exposure, Decontamination, Treatment'. https://emergency.cdc.gov/agent/cyanide/basics/facts.asp, retrieved September 9, 2023). Alitubeera, Phoebe H. P., Patricia Eyu, Benon Kwesiga, Alex R. Ario, & Bao-Ping Zhu. 'Outbreak of Cyanide Poisoning Caused by Consumption of Cassava Flour — Kasese District, Uganda, September 2017'. *Morbidity and Mortality Weekly Report (MMWR)* 68(13): 308–311. The Lucayans used cassava juice to commit suicide and avoid slavery.

44 'Governor John Gregory to Earl Grey. Support of the Poor'. The Bahamas Blue Book Report for 1849: paragraphs 192–205.

45 The Asylum Rules, tweaked again in 1879, allowed for the superintendent to put inmates to work if they were capable. Some were assigned to the laundry, while others tended a vegetable garden. 'Rules and Regulations for the New Providence Asylum'. *The Nassau Guardian,* September 20, 1879. Its staff complement is listed in Appendix 8.

46 Rosenberg, Charles E. 'Social Class and Medical Care in Nineteenth-Century America: The Rise and Fall of the Dispensary'. In *Explaining Epidemics and Other Studies in the History of Medicine.* Cambridge University Press, 1992.

47 'Public Dispensary'. The Bahamas Blue Book Report for 1851.

48 McHattie, Hon. Dr. 'Instructions to Out Island Commissioners in the Use of Medicine Supplied and in the Treatment of Certain Cases of Illness in the Absence of a Medical Man'. Bahamas Department of Archives, 1926.

49 Adderley, Rosanne Marion. *New Negroes from Africa: Slave Trade Abolition and Free African Settlement in the Nineteenth-Century Caribbean.* Indiana University Press, 2006.

50 *Ibid.*

51 'Act 13th Victoria Chapter 21. An Act to Provide for the Appointment of a Board of Health and for Otherwise Securing the Health of the Inhabitants of the Colony. Assented by the Governor'. *Bahama Herald,* April 19, 1850.

52 Fee, Elizabeth & Theodore Brown. 'The Public Health Act of 1848'. *Bulletin of the World Health Organization* 83(11) (November 2005): 866–867.

53 Brockington, Fraser. 'Public Health at The Privy Council 1805–6'. *Medical History* 7 (January 1963): 13–31.

54 'Government Notice'. *The Nassau Guardian,* May 1, 1850.

55 'Board of Health Notice'. *Bahama Herald,* June 19, 1850.

56 'Letter to The Editor from "Not One of the Board of Health"'. *Bahama Herald,* June 22, 1850.

57 The Bahamas Blue Book Report for 1851: paragraph 73.

58 Fowler, Kelly. 'A History of King's College School, Nassau, The Bahamas'. *Journal of The Bahamas Historical Society* 43 (October 2021): 16–22.

59 The Bahamas Blue Book Report for 1849.

60 'Board of Education Notice'. *Bahama Herald,* February 26, 1851.

61 'Board of Education Report to the House of Assembly'. March 19, 1853.

62 'Government Notice'. *The Nassau Guardian,* May 10, 1851. Black was trained as a surgeon and not a physician. Consequently, he was sometimes referred to as Mr, and not Dr, Black.

63 Hillside House is now the home of Majestic Tours. Saunders, D. Gail and Linda M. Huber. *Nassau's Historic Landmarks.* MacMillan, 2001.

64 Administration of Justice Colonies, &c.), 'A "Return of Judicial officers, law offices of the Crown, and other principal officers connected with the Administration of Justice in the colonies, and in India; specifying the number and descriptions of such offices, and the salaries attached to each."' June 7, 1858. Part I. North American Colonies. No 10 – Bahamas. Ordered by the House of Commons to be printed.

65 'Letter to the Editor'. *Bahama Herald,* May 15, 1850.

66 'Proceedings of the House of Assembly'. *The Nassau Guardian,* March 8, 1852.

67 'Government Notice'. *The Nassau Guardian,* May 22, 1852.

68 'Report of the Board of Health'. *The Nassau Guardian,* May 22, 1852.

69 Craton, Michael. *A History of the Bahamas.* Collins, 1968: 210.
70 Personal communication from the archivist, The King's School, Canterbury. 'History & Heritage', www.kings-school.co.uk/about/history/#slide3, retrieved March 28, 2021.
71 Wettenhall, R. L. 'Gregory, John (1795–1853)'. *Australian Dictionary of Biography,* Volume 1, 1966, https://adb.anu.edu.au/biography/gregory-john-2123, retrieved March 28, 2021.
72 Governor Gregory's salary comprised £800 from the treasury of the colony and £1,200 from Great Britain. The Bahamas Blue Book Report for 1849: paragraph 79.
73 'The Arrival of Governor Gregory'. *The Nassau Guardian,* March 3, 1849.
74 The government paid clergy a salary that ranged from £150 per annum for the rector of St Peter's, Abaco to £273 for the rector of Christ Church (The Bahamas Blue Book Report for 1849).
75 'Address of the Clergy. To His Excellency John Gregory, Esquire. Governor and Commander-in-Chief in and over the Bahama Islands, Chancellor, Vice-Admiral, and Ordinary of the Same'. *The Nassau Guardian,* March 7, 1849.
76 The Bahamas Blue Book Report for 1851.
77 'Editorial'. *Bahama Herald,* February 5, 1851.
78 'Address of the House of Assembly'. *Bahama Herald,* February 19, 1851.
79 Executive Council Minutes, October 5, 1852.
80 'Governor's Despatch'. Bahamas Department of Archives, CO23/140.
81 'Letter to the Governor from the Inhabitants'. *The Nassau Guardian,* April 10, 1852.
82 Trainor, John. 'The Ascendancy of Charles Rogers Nesbitt: Politician, Civil Servant, Administrator'. *Journal of the Bahamas Historical Society,* 3(1) (1981): 3–12.
83 'Government Notice'. *The Nassau Guardian,* July 3, 1852.
84 'C. R. Nesbitt, Lieutenant-Governor'. The Bahamas Blue Book Report for 1851.

## Notes to Chapter 2

85 Guillaume, Yodeline, Max Raymond, Gregory J. Jerome, Ralph Ternier & Louise C. Ivers. '"It Was a Ravage!": Lived Experiences of Epidemic Cholera in Rural Haiti'. *British Medical Journal of Global Health* 4(6) (2019): DOI 10.1136/bmjgh-2019-001834.
86 United Nations. 'Secretary-General Apologizes for United Nations Role in Haiti Cholera Epidemic, Urges International Funding of New Response to Disease'. UN Press Release SG/SM/18323-GA/11862, December 1, 2016, www.un.org/press/en/2016/sgsm18323.doc.htm, retrieved September 11, 2023.
87 I personally examined this patient as a consulting physician.
88 Dormandy, Thomas. *The White Death: A History of Tuberculosis.* Hambledon Press, 1999.
89 Dewhurst, Kenneth (ed.). 'A Dysentery'. In *Dr. Thomas Sydenham (1624–1689): His Life and Original Writings.* UCLA Press, 1966.
90 *Ibid.,* p. 55.
91 Osler, William. 'Cholera Asiatica'. *The Principles and Practice of Medicine,* 3rd edition. D. Appleton and Company, 1898.
92 Snow, John. *On the Mode of Communication of Cholera,* 2nd edition. Churchill, 1855.
93 Tognotti, Eugenia. 'Lessons from the History of Quarantine, from Plague to Influenza A'. *Emerging Infectious Diseases* 19(2) (2013): 254–259.
94 Howard-Jones, Norman. *The Scientific Background of the International Sanitary Conferences* 1851–1938. World Health Organization, 1975. See chapters 'The Second Conference Paris, 1859' (p. 17) and 'The Third Conference: Constantinople, 1866' (pp. 23–25).
95 Feachem, Richard, David J. Bradley, Hemda Garelick & D. Duncan Mara. '*Vibrio cholerae* and Cholera'. *Sanitation and Disease: Health Aspects of Excreta and Wastewater Management.* John Wiley & Sons, 1983.
96 *Merck's 1899 Manual of the Materia Medica together with a Summary of Therapeutic*

*Indications and a Classification of Medicaments.* Merck & Co., 1899. From a first edition of fewer than 200 pages, the twentieth edition has ballooned to over 3,500 pages.

97 Ruxin, Joshua N. 'Magic Bullet: The History of Oral Rehydration Therapy'. Medical History 38 (1994): 363–397.

98 Rosenberg, Charles E. *The Cholera Years: The United States in 1832, 1849 and 1866.* University of Chicago Press, 1962: 21–23.

99 Kiple, Kenneth F. *The Cambridge World History of Human Disease.* Cambridge University Press, 1993: 646.

100 Baly, William & William Gull. 'Reports on Epidemic Cholera Drawn up at the Desire of the Cholera Committee of the Royal College of Physicians'. John Churchill, 1854, https://wellcomecollection.org/works/uvrhvtfv/items, retrieved October 11, 2023.

101 Rosenberg, Charles E. *The Cholera Years: The United States in 1832, 1849 and 1866.* University of Chicago Press, 1962: 101–110.

102 'Letter to the Editor'. *Bahama Herald,* May 15, 1849.

103 Rosenberg, Charles E. 'Religion, Science and Progress'. In *The Cholera Years: The United States in 1832, 1849, and 1866.* University of Chicago Press, 1962: 121–132.

104 Kiple, Kenneth. F. 'Cholera and Race in the Caribbean'. *Journal of Latin American Studies* 17 (1985): 157–177.

105 Milroy, Gavin. *Cholera in Jamaica.* House of Commons, 1852: 34–35.

106 Seacole, Mary. *The Wonderful Adventures of Mrs. Seacole in Many Lands.* James Blackwood, 1857.

107 'Copies or Extracts of Despatches and Other Documents Relating to the Outbreak of Cholera in Jamaica and Respecting any Applications Made to Her Majesty's Government for the Adoption of Measures to Meet the Difficulties thus Brought upon the Colony'. House of Commons Accounts and Papers, Vol. 60. XXXVI. 561, 1851.

108 Jones, Margaret. 'Medical Services in the Immediate Post-Emancipation Period'. *Public Health in Jamaica 1850–1940: Neglect, Philanthropy and Development.* University of the West Indies Press, 2013.

109 'Parkin, John (1801–1886)'. Plarr's Lives of the Fellows, Royal College of Surgeons of England, https://livesonline.rcseng.ac.uk/client/en_GB/lives, retrieved October 2, 2022.

110 Parkin, John. *The Prevention and Treatment of Disease in the Potato and other Crops.* W. Wood, 1847.

111 Parkin, John. Statistical Report on Cholera in Jamaica. Highley and Son, 1852: 3.

112 'Copies or Extracts of Despatches and Other Documents Relating to the Outbreak of Cholera in Jamaica and Respecting any Applications Made to Her Majesty's Government for the Adoption of Measures to Meet the Difficulties thus Brought upon the Colony'. House of Commons Accounts and Papers, Vol. 60. XXXVI. 561, 1851.

113 Milroy, Gavin. *Quarantine and the Plague.* Samuel Highley, 1846.

114 Downs, Jim. *Maladies of Empire: How Colonialism, Slavery, and War Transformed Medicine.* The Belknap Press of Harvard University Press, 2021.

115 Dr Laidlaw's first name could not be found.

116 Dalrymple, Theodore. 'On the Detection of Fakes'. *British Medical Journal* 334(7599) (2007): 905.

117 Gavin, Hector. *Sanitary Ramblings. Being Sketches and Illustrations of Bethnal Green. A Type of the Condition of the Metropolis and Other Large Towns.* J. Churchill, 1848: 114–115.

118 Majer, Gerald. 'A Perfectly Beastly State of Filth: Hector Gavin, Sanitary Ramblings and the Abominable I'. *The Yale Review* 100(4) (2012): 88–113.

119 Spriggs, Edmund A. 'Hector Gavin, MD, FRCSE (1815–1855): His Life, His Work for the Sanitary Movement, and His Accidental Death in Crimea'. *Medical History* 28 (1984): 283–292.

120 Hawes, B. 'Copies or Extracts of Despatches and Other Documents Relating to the Outbreak of Cholera in the Island of Jamaica and Respecting Any Applications Made to

Her Majesty's Government for the Adoption of Measures to Meet the Difficulties Thus Brought upon the Colony. Instructions to Medical Officers Proceeding to the West Indies'. The Colonial Office, January 1, 1851. House of Commons Accounts and Papers, Vol. 6: 44–46.

121 'Medical News. Dr Hector Gavin at Bahama'. *The Lancet*, January 1, 1853.

122 Milroy, Gavin. 'The Report on the Cholera in Jamaica and on the General Sanitary Condition and Wants of the Island', enclosed in *Cholera (Jamaica): Return to an Address of the Honourable the House of Commons*, dated 20 February 1854, for a "Copy of the Report Made by Dr. Milroy to the Colonial Office, on the Cholera Epidemic in Jamaica, 1850–1851, and Copies of Extracts of Despatches Addressed to and Received from the Governor of Jamaica in Relation to the Said Report" ([1852] House of Commons, 1854), 4–109. George Edward Eyre and William Spottiswoode for HMSO, 1853, 44.

123 'Notification of the Central Board of Health. Jamaica, April 1854'. *The Barbadian*, July 28, 1854, British Library, EAP1251/1/29/6/1, https://eap.bl.uk/archive-file/EAP1251-1-29-6-1, retrieved September 11, 2023.

124 On June 6, 2023, Bella Montoya, a seventy-six-year-old retired nurse in Ecuador, narrowly escaped this fate when, hours after she had been pronounced dead of a stroke, mourners heard her banging on her coffin.

125 Bondeson, Jan. *Buried Alive: The Terrifying History of Our Most Primal Fear.* W. W. Norton & Company, 2001.

126 Park, M. P. 'Fear and Humour in the Art of Cholera'. *Journal of the Royal Society of Medicine* 103(12) (2010): 481–483. Wiertz, Antoine Joseph. *The Premature Burial* (1854). Wiertz Museum.

127 Washington, Harriet. 'Caged Subjects: Research on Black Prisoners'. In *Medical Apartheid: The Dark History of Medical Experimentation on Black Americans from Colonial Times to the Present.* Anchor Books, 2008: 266–270.

128 Downs, Jim. 'Crowded Places'. *In Maladies of Empire: How Colonialism, Slavery and War Transformed Medicine.* The Belknap Press of Harvard University Press, 2021: 26–32.

129 Milroy, *Report*, 44.

130 *Ibid.*, 44.

131 *Ibid.*, 99.

132 Jones, Norman Howard. *The Scientific Background of the International Sanitary Conferences* 1851–1938. World Health Organization, 1975: 7–11. A second Conference was held in Paris in 1859 and over the next forty years the location was rotated: Constantinople (1866), Vienna (1874), Washington, DC (1881), Rome (1885), Venice (1892), Dresden (1893) and Venice (1897). At each meeting, cholera was the main or the sole subject of discussion. In 1903, the Conference returned to Paris and remained there in the years 1911–1912, 1926 and 1938. It laid the groundwork for international health cooperation that led to the founding of the United Nations body the World Health Organization (WHO).

133 Milroy, Gavin. The International Quarantine Conference of Paris in 1851–2: with Remarks by Milroy Gavin. 1859.

## Notes to Chapter 3

135 Evans' first name remained a mystery until it was found in Talbot Bethell's 1937 book *The Early Settlers of the Bahamas and Colonists of North America.* Rounce & Wortley, 1937.

136 'Shipping Intelligence'. *The Nassau Guardian,* May 3, 1852.

137 'Shipping Intelligence'. *The Nassau Guardian,* July 14, 1852.

138 Appropriation Books of the Mercantile Navy Lists, Official Numbers 39401–39450 (39422), https://crewlist.org.uk/data/appropriation/39422, retrieved April 11, 2021.

Courtesy of nautical historian Eric Wiberg.
139 'Shipping Intelligence'. *The Nassau Guardian,* September 8, 1852.
140 Chipman, H. N. 'Cause of the Outbreak of Cholera in The Bahamas. Letter from H. N. Chipman MD, to the Editor'. *Association Medical Journal* 1(15) (1853): 335.
141 Christ Church Register of Births and Baptisms, Nassau, 1793. Courtesy of Ann Carmel.
142 Bahamas Slave Registers, 1831. Bahamas Department of Archives.
143 'Immigrant Ships Transcribers Guild: Brigantine Victoria'. Immigrantships.net, https://immigrantships.net/v13/1800v13/victoria18520618.html, retrieved June 30, 2023.
144 'Arrival of the Victoria from New York'. *Bahama Herald,* March 5, 1851.
145 Chipman, H. N. 'Cause of the Outbreak of Cholera in The Bahamas. Letter from H. N. Chipman MD, to the Editor'. *Association Medical Journal* 1(15) (1853): 335.
146 'Death Notice'. *Bahama Herald,* September 18, 1852.
147 Mrs Hall and child returned to Nassau from Harbour Island aboard the schooner Clyde. 'Shipping Intelligence'. *Bahama Herald,* September 18, 1852.
148 Farre, Frederick J. 'Cholera in The Bahamas'. *Medical Times and Gazette* 6 (1853): 300–301.
149 Chipman, H. N. and Cogswell, C. 'Cholera in the Bahamas'. *Association Medical Journal* 1(2) (1853): 46.
150 'Death Notice'. *The Nassau Guardian*, September 25, 1852.
151 'Death Notice'. *Bahama Herald,* September 25, 1852.
152 'Death Notice'. *Bahama Herald,* October 20, 1852.
153 'Editorial'. *Bahama Herald,* September 22, 1852.
154 'Editorial'. *The Nassau Guardian,* September 22, 1852.
155 The full title is 'Modern Domestic Medicine, or, A Popular Treatise, Illustrating the Character, Symptoms, Causes, Distinction, And Correct Treatment of All Diseases Incident to the Human Frame; Embracing All the Modern Improvements in Medicine With the Opinions of The Most Distinguished Physicians to Which is Added a Domestic Materia Medica; A Description of the Virtues and Correct Manner of Using the Different Mineral Waters of Europe, and the Cold, Warm, and Vapour Baths; A Copious Collection of Approved Prescriptions Adapted to Domestic Use; Ample Rules of Diet, and a Table of the Doses of Medicines, the Whole Intended as a Medical Guide for the Use of Clergymen, Heads of Families, and Invalids. Thomas John Graham, MD. Member of the Royal College of Surgeons, &c'.
156 Battley's Sedative Solution was a proprietary preparation of opium and alcohol. Laudanum was a medicine of the same main ingredients – opium and alcohol.
157 Extract from *Modern Domestic Medicine* in *The Nassau Guardian,* September 22, 1852.
158 *Ibid.*
159 Chipman, H. N. and Cogswell, C. 'Cholera in the Bahamas'. *Association Medical Journal* 1(2) (1853): 46.
160 Captain Hall returned to Nassau from Philadelphia via George Town, South Carolina on September 25. 'Shipping Intelligence'. *The Nassau Guardian,* September 29, 1852.
161 'Death Notice'. *The Nassau Guardian,* October 27, 1852.
162 'Death Notice'. *The Nassau Guardian,* November 3, 1852.
163 'Government Notice'. *The Nassau Guardian,* September 25, 1852.
164 Executive Council Minutes, September 21, 1852.
165 *Ibid.*, author's emphasis.
166 'Board of Health Notice'. *The Nassau Guardian,* September 25, 1852.
167 Bethell, A. Talbot. *The Early Settlers of the Bahamas and Colonists of North America.* Rounce & Wortley, 1937.
168 *Ibid.*
169 'Board of Health Notice'. *The Nassau Guardian.* October 9, 1852.
170 Chipman, H. N. 'Cause of the Outbreak of Cholera in The Bahamas. Letter from H.N.

Chipman MD, to the Editor'. *Association Medical Journal* 1(15) (1853): 335.
171 Bethell, A. Talbot. *The Early Settlers of the Bahamas and Colonists of North America.* Rounce & Wortley, 1937.
172 'Government Notice'. *The Nassau Guardian,* October 6, 1852.
173 'Shipping Intelligence'. *The Nassau Guardian,* September 29, 1852.
174 In 1853, Captain Dorritie sought compensation from the government for his lost shipment. His plea and the related correspondence wound up in the public record: 'Petition from Robert Dorritie, Master of the Pedraza, to the House of Assembly'. *The Nassau Guardian,* March 23, 1853.
175 *The Nassau Guardian,* March 23, 1853.
176 By contrast, the Bahamas Covid-19 epidemic produced zero deaths in the first two weeks. The thirty-fourth death from the disease came twenty-two weeks and two days after the first confirmed case. Personal communication. Dr Blair Woodside, Department of Epidemiology, Ministry of Health, The Bahamas, January 1, 2022.
177 Executive Council Minutes, September 28, 1852.
178 'Government Notice'. *The Nassau Guardian,* October 31, 1849.
179 'Advertisment'. *Bahama Herald,* May 11, 1853.
180 Executive Council Minutes, October 5, 1852. Bahamas Department of Archives
181 *Ibid.*
182 'Editorial'. *The Nassau Guardian,* October 6, 1852.
183 Paragraph 187, 'Education', in *The Reports Made to the Secretary of State Having the Department of the Colonies; in Continuation of the Reports Annually Made by the Governors of the British Colonies, With a View to Exhibit Generally The Past and Present State of Her Majesty's Colonial Possessions: Bahamas Report for 1849.* The Bahamas Department of Archives.
184 Sands, Kirkley C. *The Anglican Church and Education in The Bahamas.* The Nassau Guardian Limited, 2007; The Bahamas Blue Book Report for 1839: 142.
185 Saunders, Gail. *Bahamian Society after Emancipation.* MacMillan Caribbean, 2003.
186 'Notice: The Sale of Pews'. *Bahama Herald,* May 11, 1853.
187 Turner, Grace. *Honoring Ancestors in Sacred Space: The Archaeology of an Eighteenth-Century African-Bahamian Cemetery.* University Press of Florida, 2017.
188 Thompson, Gilbert. 'The Burial Ground Controversy'. In *A Goodly Heritage: A Concise History of the Diocese of The Bahamas and The Turks and Caicos Islands.* 12 Avenue Graphics, 2012, 173–176.
189 'An Act for Defining the Right to the Ceremonial Use of Certain Burial Grounds in the Island of New Providence'. 13 Victoria Ch. 5. March 14, 1850.
190 'Editorial'. *Bahama Herald,* January 29, 1851.
191 'Charge of the Lord Bishop of Jamaica to his Clergy in the Bahamas'. *Bahama Herald,* April 2, 1850.
192 'Proceedings of the House of Assembly'. *The Nassau Guardian,* March 3, 1852.
193 'Government Notice'. *The Nassau Guardian,* October 9, 1852.
194 *Ibid.*
195 McWeeney, Sean. *Breaching the Gates: The Bahamian Free Coloured and the Struggle for Civil Rights 1802–1834.* Sean McWeeney, 2018; 'Death Notice'. *The Nassau Guardian,* October 17, 1857.
196 'Petition from James Ross to Governor Gregory and Letters of Support from Reverends J. S. Hildebrand, Henry MacDougall, Isaac Whitehouse and William Maclure'. *The Nassau Guardian,* March 26, 1853.
197 Executive Council Minutes, October 9, 1852.
198 'Government Notice'. *The Nassau Guardian,* October 13, 1852.
199 'Government Notice'. *The Nassau Guardian,* October 16, 1852.
200 *Ibid.*

201 Executive Council Minutes, October 11, 1852.
202 'Government Notice'. *The Nassau Guardian,* October 16, 1852.
203 'Editorial'. *The Nassau Guardian,* October 13, 1852: 2.
204 'Government Notice'. *Bahama Herald,* October 16, 1852.
205 MH 13/248, British National Archives.
206 The surviving portion of Charles Farquharson's journal, 1831–1832, describes the day-to-day operation of his slave plantation on Watlings Island. The original is in the custody of the Bahamas Department of Archives.
207 Farquharson collection. Bahamas Department of Archives.
208 'Editorial'. *The Nassau Guardian,* November 3, 1852.

## Notes to Chapter 4

209 'Editorial'. *The Nassau Guardian,* November 10, 1852.
210 *The Nassau Guardian's* account mentions just one daughter in the travelling party. Hector Gavin's account reports that the party included the His Excellency's 'two adult daughters'. Neither account mentions the baby born to the governor and Mrs Gregory in Government House on February 2, 1851.
211 Entry for the RMS *Esk* on the Ships List, www.theshipslist.com/ships/descriptions/ShipsE.shtml, retrieved August 17, 2022.
212 'Editorial'. *The Nassau Guardian,* April 2, 1853.
213 *Sorrow on the Sea: Being an Account of the Loss of the Steam-Ship "Amazon" by Fire.* J. Mason, 1852.
214 'Letter from Dr Gavin to the Right Hon. Earl Desart. Nassau, New Providence, January 1853'; 'Copies or Extracts from Despatches from the Governor of Barbadoes, Respecting the Admission of Her Majesty's Ship "Dauntless" to Free Pratique in the Island'; and 'Letter from Dr Gavin, Stating Certain Facts in Connexion with Yellow Fever on Board the Steam Packet "Esk," while at Nassau'. House of Commons, March 18, 1853.
215 'Governor's Despatch to Pakington, December 4, 1852'. CO 23/140, Bahamas Department of Archives.
216 *Ibid.*
217 Gavin to Gregory, November 8, 1852. MH 13/248, British National Archives.
218 'Vincent Burial'. *The Nassau Guardian,* November 10, 1852.
219 CO 23/140, Bahamas Department of Archives.
220 *Ibid*
221 The question of quarantine was finally settled in 1900, when it was proved that yellow fever was transmitted by mosquitoes and not from person to person.
222 CO 23/140, Bahamas Department of Archives.
223 Rosenberg, Charles E. *The Cholera Years: The United States in 1832, 1849, and 1866.* University of Chicago Press, 1962: 59.
224 CO 23/140, Bahamas Department of Archives.
225 'Hector Gavin to the Earl of Desart, November 11, 1852'. MH 13/248, British National Archives.
226 'Death Notice'. *The Nassau Guardian,* November 20, 1852.
227 'General Court'. *The Nassau Guardian,* October 30, 1852.
228 MH 13/248, British National Archives.
229 The Nuisances Removal and Diseases Prevention Act 1846.
230 Executive Council Minutes, November 10, 1852.
231 The Nuisances Removal and Diseases Prevention Act 1846 was meant to be temporary legislation to help to stem the spread of cholera in England. The Health Foundation Policy Navigator. 'The Nuisances Removal and Diseases Prevention Act 1846',

https://navigator.health.org.uk/theme/nuisances-removal-and-diseases-prevention-act-1846, retrieved August 16, 2021.
232 Executive Council Minutes, November 10, 1852.
233 'Notice of Resignation'. *The Nassau Guardian,* November 20, 1852.
234 'Letter to Drs Kirkwood, Chipman and Duncome from his Excellency the Governor'. *The Nassau Guardian,* November 20, 1852.
235 Dr Hector Gavin to his Excellency the Governor. Executive Council Minutes, November 16, 1852.
236 Letter from Drs Kirkwood, Chipman and Duncome to his Excellency the Governor. Executive Council Minutes, November 16, 1852.
237 *Ibid.*
238 'Board of Health Notice. New Health Districts'. *The Nassau Guardian,* November 24, 1853, emphasis original.
239 'Abstract of Returns from the Board of Health'. *The Nassau Guardian,* November 20, 1852.
240 'Returns of Deaths from Cholera and Other Causes'. *The Nassau Guardian,* November 24, 1852.
241 'Editorial'. *The Nassau Guardian,* November 17, 1852.
242 'Shipping Intelligence'. *The Nassau Guardian,* November 20, 1852.
243 'Board of Health Notice'. *The Nassau Guardian,* November 27, 1852.
244 'Board of Health Notice: Hospital Accommodation'. *The Nassau Guardian,* November 24, 1852.
245 Farre, Frederick J. 'Cholera in The Bahamas'. *Medical Times and Gazette* 6 (1853): 300–301.
246 'John Richard Farre'. Royal College of Physicians, https://history.rcplondon.ac.uk/inspiring-physicians/john-richard-farre, retrieved 12 September 2023.
247 'Arthur Farre'. Royal College of Physicians, https://history.rcplondon.ac.uk/inspiring-physicians/arthur-farre, retrieved 12 September 2023.
248 'Frederick Farre'. Royal College of Physicians, https://history.rcplondon.ac.uk/inspiring-physicians/frederic-john-farre, retrieved 12 September 2023.
249 Russell, Richard. *A Dissertation Concerning the Use of Sea Water in Diseases of the Glands etc. to Which is Added an Epistolary Dissertation to R. Frewin.* Fletcher and Rivington, 1753.
250 'Margate's Sea Bathing Hospital'. Historic Hospitals, https://historic-hospitals.com/2017/12/27/margates-sea-bathing-hospital/, retrieved June 8, 2022.
251 'Letter to the Editor'. *Bahama Herald,* August 13, 1853.
252 *Ibid.*
253 'Government Notices'. *The Nassau Guardian,* September 1, 4 and 8, 1852.
254 Farre, Frederick John. 'Cholera in The Bahamas'. *Medical Times and Gazette* 6 (1853): 300–301.
255 'Board of Health Notice'. *The Nassau Guardian,* November 20, 1852.
256 Farre, Frederick J. 'Cholera in The Bahamas'. *Medical Times and Gazette* 6 (1853): 300–301.
257 Slavery continued in the USA, Cuba and Brazil until 1865, 1886 and 1888 respectively.
258 CO 23/140, Despatch to Sir John Pakington, December 4, 1852, Bahamas Department of Archives.
259 *Ibid.*
260 *Ibid.*
261 *Ibid.*
262 *Ibid.*

## Notes to Chapter 5

263 'Editor's Letter Box. Cholera in The Bahamas: Remarks by Dr Chipman, communicated by Dr Cogswell to The Editor'. *Association Medical Journal,* January 14, 1853.
264 'Sarah Anne Chipman Obituary'. *The Nassau Guardian,* January 1, 1853.
265 'Hector Gavin M.D. Letter to the Editor'. *The Nassau Guardian,* February 5, 1853.
266 *Ibid.*
267 'Correspondence with the Board of Health and the Medical Practitioners of Nassau, Relative to the Supply of Medicines, and Medical Attendance for the Relief of the Poor, Who Might be Afflicted with Cholera in Nov. 1852'. Referred to in the Governor's message to the House of Assembly, No. 5, dated March 8, 1853. *The Nassau Guardian,* March 19, 1853.
268 Governor Gregory despatch, CO 23/140, Bahamas Department of Archives.
269 'Editorial'. *The Nassau Guardian,* November 27, 1852.
270 'Letter to the Editor'. *The Nassau Guardian,* November 24, 1852.
271 *Ibid.*
272 'Died'. *The Nassau Guardian,* December 4, 1852.
273 'Died'. *The Nassau Guardian,* January 19, 1853.
274 'Dr Clutsam Obituary'. *The Nassau Guardian,* June 25, 1853.
275 'Notice'. *Bahama Herald,* March 8, 1851.
276 CO 23/140, Despatch to Sir John Pakington, December 4, 1852, Bahamas Department of Archives.
277 'Shipping Intelligence'. *The Nassau Guardian,* November 24, 1852.
278 'Editorial: Abaco'. *The Nassau Guardian,* December 15, 1852.
279 Lawlor, Ann and Jim Lawlor. *The Harbour Island Story.* MacMillan Caribbean, 2008: 109–115.
280 *Ibid.*
281 *Ibid.*
282 Executive Council Minutes, October 15, 1852.
283 *Ibid.*
284 'Editorial'. *The Nassau Guardian,* October 23, December 18 and 22, 1852.
285 'Obituary. Editorial Department'. *Buffalo Medical Journal and Monthly Review* 8 (11) (1853): 719.
286 'Dr Benjamin Wendel Obituary'. *Bahama Herald,* May 11, 1853.
287 Catalogue of the Trustees, Officers & Students of the University of Pennsylvania, Session 1850–1851.
288 'Editorial'. *The Nassau Guardian,* November 20, 1852.
289 'Death of Dr B. F. Wendel'. *Bahama Herald,* May 11, 1853.
290 'Editorial'. *The Nassau Guardian,* November 20, 1852.
291 The cause of Eliza's demise, contrary to the usual practice, was pointedly omitted from her death notice in *The Nassau Guardian,* December 22, 1852.
292 Lawlor, Jim. *Paul Albury: A Man and His Writings.* Media Enterprises Ltd, 2013: 27.
293 Catalogue of the alumni of the Medical Department of the University of Pennsylvania, 1765–1877. US National Library of Medicine, https://collections.nlm.nih.gov/catalog/nlm:nlmuid-26821300R-bk, retrieved September 13, 2021.
294 'Married'. *Bahama Herald,* February 11, 1860.
295 Dr Johnson's son, A. T. W. Johnson, followed him into the medical profession. His grandson, Hugh Johnson, was a dentist and mentor to Paul Albury, a Harbour Island native, McGill graduate in dentistry and, in the 1970s, a noted Bahamian historian.
296 'Cholera Panic in Eleuthera'. *The Nassau Guardian,* December 1, 1852; CO 23/140: 234, Bahamas Department of Archives.

297 'Proclamation'. *The Nassau Guardian*, December 4, 1852
298 'Editorial'. *The Nassau Guardian,* December 22, 1852.
299 'Letter to the Editor'. T*he Nassau Guardian,* December 11, 1852.
300 'Government Notice'. *The Nassau Guardian,* December 18, 1852.

## Notes to Chapter 6

301 'News from Havre, September 29'. *Charleston Courier,* October 15, 1852.
302 'Immigration to the United States, 1851–1900'. Library of Congress, www.loc.gov/classroom-materials/united-states-history-primary-source-timeline/rise-of-industrial-america-1876-1900/immigration-to-united-states-1851-1900/, retrieved August 29, 2021.
303 Woodham-Smith, Cecil. *The Great Hunger: Ireland 1845–1849.* Penguin Books, 1991: 206–217.
304 Zimmermann, Gotthelf. 'Auswanderer-Karte und Wegweiser nach Nordamerika' ['Emigrant's Map and Guide for Routes to North America']. J. B. Metzlerschen Buchhandlung, 1853. The World Digital Library, www.wdl.org/en/item/41/, retrieved August 23, 2021.
305 Lawlor, Jim. 'Wrecked Emigrant Ships in The Bahamas: The Wreck of the Barque *William and Mary*'. *International Journal of Bahamian Studies* 27 (2021). https://doi.org/10.15362/ijbs.v27i0.411.
306 'Editorial'. *The Nassau Guardian,* December 4, 1852.
307 Executive Council Minutes, September 21, 1852.
308 *Royal Gazette,* December 8, 1852, quoted in the *Charleston Courier,* December 23, 1852.
309 'Coroner's Inquest'. *The Nassau Guardian,* December 8, 1852.
310 *Ibid.*
311 'A. T. Holmes Notice'. *The Nassau Guardian,* December 15, 1852.
312 'Letter to the Editor'. *The Nassau Guardian,* December 11, 1852.
313 The Bahamas Blue Book Report for 1849: 155.
314 Governor Gregory to Sir John Pakington. CO 23/140: 254–257, Bahamas Department of Archives.
315 MacDougall, Henry. 'Letter to the Editor'. *The Nassau Guardian,* December 11, 1852.
316 'Government Notice'. *Bahama Herald,* September 25, 1852.
317 'Editorial'. *The Nassau Guardian,* December 11, 1852.
318 Thomson was appointed on July 23, 1852. 'Government Notice'. *Bahama Herald,* September 15, 1852.
319 'A Card'. *The Nassau Guardian,* December 15, 1852.
320 Symonette, Michael and Antonia Canzoneri. *Baptists in the Bahamas: An Historical Review.* Baptist Spanish Publishing House, 1977: 28–30.
321 Cox, Francis A. 'History of the Baptist Missionary Society from 1792–1842: Baptist Missionaries and Baptist Work in The Bahamas'. *The Baptist Quarterly 2* (1988): 295–297.
322 Symonette, Michael and Antonia Canzoneri. *Baptists in the Bahamas: An Historical Review.* Baptist Spanish Publishing House, 1977: 36–37.
323 'Editorial'. *The Nassau Guardian,* December 15, 1852.
324 *Ibid.*
325 'Death Notice'. *The Nassau Guardian,* December 15, 1852.
326 *Ibid.*
327 'Later [*sic*] from Nassau'. *Charleston Courier,* December 23, 1852.
328 'Death of Dr Thomas Young Simons'. *Charleston Courier,* June 9, 1857.
329 Simons, Thomas Y. 'A Report on the History and Causes of the Strangers or Yellow Fever of Charleston: Read before the Board of Health'. Charleston Board of Health, North Carolina, 1839.

330 'The Emigrant Passengers in the Brig Pedraza'. *Charleston Courier,* January 4, 1853; *Charleston Mercury,* January 7, 1853.
331 'Minutes. Meeting of the German Friendly Society, held on Wednesday Evening, December 29th, 1852'. *Journal of the German Friendly Society.* Special Collections Archives, South Carolina Historical Society.
332 City of Charleston Health Department Death Records, January 1846 through December 1852. Charleston Public Library.
333 Waring, Joseph Ioor. 'Asiatic Cholera in South Carolina'. *Bulletin of the History of Medicine* 60(5) (1966): 459–466.
334 'Letter from Mnsr. Fogt, Translated from French'. *The Nassau Guardian,* February 12, 1853.
335 'Letter from Theodore Strempel, Translated from German'. *The Nassau Guardian,* February 16, 1853.
336 'Editorial'. *The Nassau Guardian,* December 25, 1852.
337 'Shipping Intelligence'. *The Nassau Guardian,* January 1, 1853.
338 'Minutes, City Commissioners Meeting'. *Charleston Daily Courier,* January 5, 1853.

## Notes to Chapter 7

339 'Election Notices'. The Nassau Guardian, January 5, 1853.
340 Farre, Frederick J. 'Cholera in The Bahamas'. Medical Times and Gazette 6 (1853): 300–301.
341 'Election Results'. The Nassau Guardian, January 8, 1853.
342 'Church Missionary Hall'. The Nassau Guardian, January 12, 1853.
343 'A Bazaar'. Bahama Herald, May 11, 1853.
344 'Bahama Board of Health Notice'. The Nassau Guardian, January 5, 1853.
345 Pemberton, Rita. 'Dirt, Disease and Death: Control, Resistance and Change in the Post-Emancipation Caribbean'. Historia, Ciencias, Saude 19 (suppl. December 2012): 47–58.
346 Executive Council Minutes, January 3, 1853.
347 Ibid.
348 Executive Council Minutes, January 17, 1853.
349 Ibid.
350 Ibid.
351 The author has not been able to locate this letter, which was said to have come out in November 1852.
352 'Pamphlets: 1. The Unhealthiness of London. 2. Habitations of the Industrial Classes; their Physical, Social and Moral Influence'. The Nassau Guardian, January 22, 1853.
353 Executive Council Minutes, February 2, 1853.
354 Exact amount was £317.11s.4½d.
355 'Letter to the Editor'. The Nassau Guardian, February 5, 1853. Full text of the letter appears in Appendix 3.
356 Ibid.
357 'Shipping Intelligence'. The Nassau Guardian, February 9, 1853.
358 'The Governor's speech to the President and Gentlemen of the Legislative Council and the Speaker and Gentlemen of the House of Assembly. Opening of the Legislature'. The Nassau Guardian, February 23, 1853.
359 The receiver recorded £26,104 in 1852 compared to £24,273 in the previous year. Ibid.
360 Proceedings of the House of Assembly, March 16, 1853.
361 Josey, Arnold E. The Story of Baptists in the Bahamas: An Historical Survey. Xulon Press, 2015: 66–67.
362 'Rum Cay'. The Nassau Guardian, December 11, 1852.

363 Symonette, Michael and Antonia Canzoneri. Baptists in the Bahamas: An Historical Review. Baptist Spanish Publishing House, 1977: 36.
364 'Proclamation'. The Nassau Guardian, February 12, 1853.
365 'The Hon. House of Assembly. Documents Referred to In minutes of the 5th April 1853, Relating to the Seizure by the Revenual Officers of Certain Goods Consigned to the Rev'd. Henry Capern'. The Nassau Guardian, April 13, 1853.
366 The force landed and discovered that it was not needed. In December, the Treaty of Ghent had been signed and news finally arrived that the war was over. Caulfield, James E. 100 Years' History of the 2nd West India Regiment: 1795–1892. Andrews, 2011: 35.
367 Clerk of the House. '41st Conference of the Commonwealth Parliament Association'. The Bahamas Government, https://t.ly/Th7q5, retrieved May 12, 2022.
368 'John Grant Anderson'. WikiTree, www.wikitree.com/wiki/Anderson-38379, retrieved May 2, 2022.
369 'House of Assembly. Documents Referred to in Minutes of the 5th April 1853, Relating to the Seizure by the Revenual Officers of Certain Goods Consigned to the Rev'd Henry Capern'. The Nassau Guardian, April 13, 1853.
370 Ibid.
371 'Vere Foster, Letter to the Editor'. The Nassau Guardian, February 19, 1853.
372 'Notice Posted by Vere Foster'. The Nassau Guardian, February 16, 1853.
373 'Governor Gregory to the Duke of Newcastle'. The Bahamas Archives, May 3, 1853.
374 'Shipping Intelligence'. The Nassau Guardian, May 7, 1853.
375 'Government Notice'. The Nassau Guardian, May 4 and 7, 1853.
376 The government had just granted the young clergyman leave from St Phillips Church in order to travel to Jamaica, where he was to be promoted to the priesthood.
377 Gottlieb von Sanden, Owanta. Angel Stand by Me. Daybreak Publishing, 1987.
378 Lawlor, Jim. 'Wrecked Emigrant Ships in The Bahamas: The Wreck of the Barque William and Mary'. International Journal of Bahamian Studies 27 (2021). DOI: 10.15362/ijbs.v27i0.411.
379 Bahama Herald, May 11, 1853.
380 Capern returned to New Providence after his vacation and served until he retired in 1857. He died in Belvedere, Kent on April 12, 1883. Symonette, Michael C. and Antonina Canzoneri. Baptists in the Bahamas: An Historical Review. Baptist Spanish Publishing House, 1977.
381 J. G. Anderson died in Nassau three years later, on August 25, 1855.

## Notes to Chapter 8

382 'Despatch from Governor Gregory to Sir John Pakington'. CO 23/140, Bahamas Department of Archives.
383 Makepeace, William T. and Richard P. Dyer. Wesley Methodist Church: Souvenir of the Centenary, 1847–1947. Nassau, 1947.
384 'Board of Health Notice'. The Nassau Guardian, November 20, 1852.
385 MH 13/248: 399, British National Archives.
386 Ibid.
387 Kiple, Kenneth. F. 'Cholera and Race in the Caribbean'. Journal of Latin American Studies 17 (1985): 157–177.
388 Khalifa, Mohammed M., Radwa R. Sharaf and Ramy K. Aziz. 'Helicobacter pylori: A Poor Man's Gut Pathogen?' Gut Pathogens 2(1) (2010): 2.
389 Milroy, Gavin. 'The Report on the Cholera in Jamaica and on the General Sanitary Condition and Wants of the Island', enclosed in Cholera (Jamaica): Return to an Address of the Honourable the House of Commons, dated 20 February 1854, for a "Copy of the

Report Made by Dr. Milroy to the Colonial Office, on the Cholera Epidemic in Jamaica, 1850–1851, and Copies of Extracts of Despatches Addressed to and Received from the Governor of Jamaica in Relation to the Said Report" ([1852] House of Commons, 1854), 4–109. George Edward Eyre and William Spottiswoode for HMSO, 1853, 22.

390 In 1974, there were 1,032 deaths in The Bahamas. In 1995, the number was 1,604 deaths. Courtesy of Mr Dwayne Archer, Bahamas Department of Statistics.

391 From 26,491 in 1845 to 27,519 in 1851 and then to 35,487 in 1861. Bahamas Department of Statistics.

392 The Bahamas Blue Book Report for 1849: paragraphs 38 and 39.

393 The Bahamas Blue Book Report for 1851: paragraph 78.

394 Nobles, Jenna, Elizabeth Frankenberg and Duncan Thomas. 'The Effects of Mortality on Fertility: Population Dynamics After a Natural Disaster'. Demography 52(1) (2015): 15–18.

395 Finlay, Jocelyn. Fertility Response to Natural Disasters: The Case of Three High Mortality Earthquakes. World Bank Policy Research Working Paper No. 4883, 2009.

396 'Dr Clutsam's Bill'. The Nassau Guardian, March 23, 1853.

397 Exactly £142.16d.

398 Executive Council Minutes, March 2, 1853.

399 Executive Council Minutes, June 2, 1853.

400 'Editorial'. The Nassau Guardian, July 27, 1853.

401 'Editorial'. Bahama Herald, July 30, 1853.

402 'Opening of the Legislature'. *The Nassau Guardian,* February 7, 1855.

403 'Tenders. The Board of Public Works'. The Nassau Guardian, July 1, 1857.

404 Brooker, Colin. 'The Quarantine Station and East Ruin, Athol Island, New Providence'. Journal of the Bahamas Historical Society 30 (2008): 25–34.

405 Chipman, H. N. 'Cause of the Outbreak of Cholera in The Bahamas. Letter from H. N. Chipman MD, to the Editor'. Association Medical Journal, April 15, 1853: 335.

406 Ibid.

407 The Last Will and Testament of Horatio Chipman MD, June 13, 1873. Bahamas Department of Archives.

408 'Bahama Literary Association'. The Nassau Guardian, October 4, 1851.

409 'Notice of Dr J. F. H. Chipman'. The Nassau Guardian, January 20, 1864.

410 'Obituary of Dr H. N. Chipman'. The Nassau Guardian, July 19, 1873.

411 Chipman, Donna. Bahamian Cultural Dynasty Book 1 with 'Chippie' The Honourable John Arthur (Chippie) Chipman MBE, OMA King of the Goombay/Junkanoo Drums & Godfather of Culture. PMT Atlantean, 2001.

412 Trainor, John. 'The Ascendancy of Charles Rogers Nesbitt: Politician, Civil Servant, Administrator'. Journal of the Bahamas Historical Society 3(1) (1981): 3–12.

413 At some point in the 1860s, Dr Duncome began spelling his name 'Duncombe'.

414 'Dr Frederick Duncombe Obituary'. The Nassau Guardian, March 25, 1882.

415 The Dundee Courier, November 9, 1853.

416 Nightingale, Florence. 'Notes on Hospitals, being Two Papers Read before the National Association for the Promotion of Social Science, at Liverpool, in October, 1858: With Evidence Given to the Royal Commissioners on the State of the Army in 1857'.

417 Woodham-Smith, Cecil. Florence Nightingale: 1820–1910. Constable, 1950: 139.

418 Ibid., p. 188.

419 Spriggs, Edmund A. 'Hector Gavin MD FRCSE (1815–1855): His Life, His Work for the Sanitary Movement, and his Accidental Death in the Crimea'. Medical History 28(3) (1984): 283–292.

420 Neely, Wayne. The Greatest and Deadliest Hurricanes to Impact The Bahamas: The Stories behind the Great Storms. iUniverse, 2011; 156.

421 The Nassau Guardian, October 10, 1866.

422 'How to Avoid Fever, Consumption or Cholera: Papers on Sanitation by the Hon. W. Kirkwood MD MLC, Hon. G.T.R. Kemp MD MEC, J. B. Albury MD, W. Robinson LRCSI and Hon W. M. G. Maclure MD MLC. With an Introduction by His Excellency the Governor', 1884. CO 23/225, Bahamas Department of Archives.

423 Ibid.

424 Ibid.

425 Rosenberg, Charles E. The Cholera Years: The United States in 1832, 1849, and 1866. University of Chicago Press, 1962: 9.

426 Johnson, Steven. The Ghost Map: The Story of London's Most Terrifying Epidemic and How It Changed Science, Cities, and the Modern World. Riverhead Books, 2006.

427 'How to Avoid Fever, Consumption or Cholera: Papers on Sanitation by the Hon. W. Kirkwood MD MLC, Hon. G.T.R. Kemp MD MEC, J. B. Albury MD, W. Robinson LRCSI and Hon W. M. G. Maclure MD MLC. With an Introduction by His Excellency the Governor', 1884. CO 23/225, Bahamas Department of Archives.

428 'Abby Dickinson Kirkwood, wife of William Kirkwood MD for 52 years. Born at Hadley, Mass. April 12, 1813. Died Oct. 21, 1888'. Gravestone inscription, Western Cemetery, New Providence.

429 'Obituary'. The Nassau Guardian, December 12, 1888.

430 The Last Will and Testament of William Kirkwood MD, December 12, 1888.

431 A photograph of the beautiful home in its prime appears in Lightbourn, Ronald G. Reminiscing II: Photographs of Old Nassau. R. G. Lightbourn 2005; 117.

432 Moseley Moss, Valeria. Reminiscing: Memories of Old Nassau. R. G. Lightbourn, 1999; 106. Sir Harold Christie is known as the father of real estate business in The Bahamas. He was a one-time close friend of Sir Harry Oakes and slept at the tycoon's estate on the night of his unsolved murder in the house.

433 Personal communication with the treasurer, Christ Church Cathedral, September 2022.

434 Monteil, Charlotte, Jenni Barclay and Anna Hicks. 'Remembering, Forgetting, and Absencing Disasters in the Post-Disaster Recovery Process'. International Journal of Disaster Risk Science 11 (2020): 287–299.

435 The Barbadian, September 16, 1854, EAP1251/1/29/9/1, British Library.

436 The Barbadian, January 10, 1855, EAP 1251/1/30/1/2, British Library.

437 The Barbadian, November 22, 1854.

438 Jones, Margaret. Public Health in Jamaica 1850–1940: Neglect, Philanthropy and Development. University of the West Indies Press, 2013: 72–76.

439 Collymore-Taylor, Wayne. 'History of Water Services in Barbados 1857–2016'. https://issuu.com/waynecolly/docs/476430734-government-intervention-of-the-origin-of, retrieved January 29, 2023.

440 Hammel, Zach. 'Modernity in a Monument: Memory and the Gore Park Fountains', in Herring, D. Ann and Battles, Heather T. (eds), Ch$_2$olera: Hamilton's Forgotten Epidemics. McMaster University Anthropology Publications. Paper 6, 2012.

441 'Governor G. B. Haddon-Smith to the Secretary of State the Right Honourable Lewis Harcourt P.C.', August 21, 1913. The Bahamas Water and Sewerage Corporation Archives.

442 Ibid.

443 Humphreys, H. Howard. 'Proposed Waterworks for the City of Nassau'. Colony of The Bahamas, May 18, 1914. The Bahamas Water and Sewerage Corporation Archives.

444 'Dr A. H. B. Pearce to the Dr G. H. Johnson, Chairman of the Board of Health', July 2, 1923. Bahamas Department of Archives.

445 Beveridge, Wilfred W. O. Report of the Public Health and on Medical Conditions in New Providence, Bahama Islands. Waterlow, 1927. Bahamas Department of Archives.

446 'Mrs Frances Stoddard'. The New York Times, March 26, 1929.

447 Cruickshank, J. M. 'An Anti-Typhoid Campaign'. Perspectives in Public Health 59(2) (1938). https://doi.org/10.1177/146642403805900021.

448 Annual Reports of the Chief Medical Officer, 1963, 1965, 1973.
449 Deshpande, V. and Munnings, H. 'Amoebiasis Presenting as an Abdominal Wall Abscess (Amoeboma Cutis)'. West Indies Medical Journal 36 (1987): 108–109.
450 Swann, Michael. National Water Week, Commemorative Booklet. May 2–7, 1993. The Bahamas Water and Sewerage Corporation Archives.
451 Water Resources Assessment of The Bahamas. US Army Corp of Engineers, Mobile District and Topographic Engineering Center, 2004.
452 Poirier, Mathieu J. P., Ricardo Izurieta, Sharad S. Malavade and Michael D. MacDonald. 'Re-Emergence of Cholera in the Americas: Risks, Susceptibility and Ecology'. Journal of Global Infectious Disease 4(3) (2012): 162–171.
453 'The Yarmouth Castle Disaster' was featured on the cover of Life Magazine and inspired a song by Gordon Lightfoot. Footage of the tragedy has been uploaded to YouTube.

## Notes to Epilogue

454 'National Action on Cane Toad Underway'. Government of The Bahamas Press Release, June 2, 2020.
455 'Nearly 400 Invasive Cane Toads Caught'. The Tribune, August 7, 2020.

## Notes to Appendix 3

456 The Nuisances Removal and Diseases Prevention Act 1846 was meant to be temporary legislation to help to stem the spread of cholera in England. The Health Foundation Policy Navigator. 'The Nuisances Removal and Diseases Prevention Act 1846', https://navigator.health.org.uk/theme/nuisances-removal-and-diseases-prevention-act-1846, retrieved August 16, 2021.

## Notes to Appendix 7

457 'Ship Registers and Enrollments of New Orleans, Louisiana 1851–1860'. Family Search, www.familysearch.org/search/catalog/2364506, retrieved July 4, 2023.

# Index

www.ingramcontent.com/pod-product-compliance
Lightning Source LLC
Chambersburg PA
CBHW041258210926
51847CB00009B/64
*9789768205643*